Behavior as an Illness Indicator

Editor

ELIZABETH STELOW

VETERINARY CLINICS OF NORTH AMERICA: SMALL ANIMAL PRACTICE

www.vetsmall.theclinics.com

May 2018 • Volume 48 • Number 3

ELSEVIER

1600 John F. Kennedy Boulevard • Suite 1800 • Philadelphia, Pennsylvania, 19103-2899

http://www.vetsmall.theclinics.com

VETERINARY CLINICS OF NORTH AMERICA: SMALL ANIMAL PRACTICE Volume 48, Number 3
May 2018 ISSN 0195-5616, ISBN-13: 978-0-323-58382-4

Editor: Colleen Dietzler
Developmental Editor: Meredith Madeira

Veterinary Clinics of North America: Small Animal Practice (ISSN 0195-5616) is published bimonthly by Elsevier Inc., 360 Park Avenue South, New York, NY 10010-1710. Months of issue are January, March, May, July, September, and November. Business and Editorial Offices: 1600 John F. Kennedy Blvd., Ste. 1800, Philadelphia, PA 19103-2899. Customer Service Office: 3251 Riverport Lane, Maryland Heights, MO 63043. Periodicals postage paid at New York, NY and additional mailing offices. Subscription prices are $325.00 per year (domestic individuals), $622.00 per year (domestic institutions), $100.00 per year (domestic students/residents), $430.00 per year (Canadian individuals), $773.00 per year (Canadian institutions), $469.00 per year (international individuals), $773.00 per year (international institutions), and $220.00 per year (international and Canadian students/residents). To receive student/resident rate, orders must be accompanied by name of affiliated institution, date of term, and the *signature* of program/residency coordinator on institution letterhead. Orders will be billed at individual rate until proof of status is received. Foreign air speed delivery is included in all *Clinics* subscription prices. All prices are subject to change without notice. **POSTMASTER:** Send address changes to *Veterinary Clinics of North America: Small Animal Practice*, Elsevier Health Sciences Division, Subscription Customer Service, 3251 Riverport Lane, Maryland Heights, MO 63043. Customer Service (orders, claims, online, change of address): Elsevier Periodicals Customer Service, Elsevier Health Sciences Division Subscription **Customer Service 3251 Riverport Lane Maryland Heights, MO 63043. Tel: 1-800-654-2452 (U.S. and Canada); 314-447-8871 (outside U.S. and Canada). Fax: 314-447-8029. E-mail: journalscustomerservice-usa@elsevier.com (for print support); journalsonlinesupport-usa@elsevier.com (for online support).**

Reprints. For copies of 100 or more of articles in this publication, please contact the Commercial Reprints Department, Elsevier Inc., 360 Park Avenue South, New York, NY 10010-1710. Tel.: 212-633-3874; Fax: 212-633-3820; E-mail: reprints@elsevier.com.

Veterinary Clinics of North America: Small Animal Practice is also published in Japanese by Inter Zoo Publishing Co., Ltd., Aoyama Crystal-Bldg 5F, 3-5-12 Kitaaoyama, Minato-ku, Tokyo 107-0061, Japan.

Veterinary Clinics of North America: Small Animal Practice is covered in *Current Contents/Agriculture, Biology and Environmental Sciences, Science Citation Index, ASCA, MEDLINE/PubMed (Index Medicus), Excerpta Medica, and BIOSIS.*

Contributors

EDITOR

ELIZABETH STELOW, DVM
Diplomate, American College of Veterinary Behaviorists; Clinical Animal Behavior Service, UC Davis Veterinary Medical Teaching Hospital, Davis, California, USA

AUTHORS

KELLY C. BALLANTYNE, DVM
Diplomate, American College of Veterinary Behaviorists; Clinical Assistant Professor of Veterinary Behavior, Veterinary Clinical Medicine, University of Illinois College of Veterinary Medicine, Chicago, Illinois, USA

LETICIA MATTOS DE SOUZA DANTAS, DVM, MS, PhD
Diplomate, American College of Veterinary Behaviorists; Veterinary Educational Specialist, Behavioral Medicine Service, University of Georgia Veterinary Teaching Hospital, University of Georgia College of Veterinary Medicine, Athens, Georgia, USA

ISABELLE DEMONTIGNY-BÉDARD, DMV, MSc
Diplomate, American College of Veterinary Behaviorsts; Veterinary Behaviorist, Centre Vétérinaire DMV, Montreal, Québec, Canada

DIANE FRANK, DMV
Diplomate, American College of Veterinary Behaviorsts; Professor, Department of Clinical Sciences, Faculty of Veterinary Medicine, University of Montreal, Saint-Hyacinthe, Québec, Canada

JILLIAN M. ORLANDO, DVM
Carolina Veterinary Behavior Clinic, Raleigh, North Carolina, USA

AMY PIKE, DVM
Diplomate, American College of Veterinary Behaviorists; Behavior Medicine Division, Veterinary Referral Center of Northern Virginia, Manassas, Virginia, USA

SABRINA POGGIAGLIOLMI, DVM, MS
Diplomate, American College of Veterinary Behaviorists; Long Island Veterinary Specialists, Plainview, New York, USA

ERANDA RAJAPAKSHA, BVSc, MS, PhD
Diplomate, American College of Veterinary Behaviorists; Diplomate, American College of Animal Welfare; Department of Veterinary Clinical Sciences, University of Peradeniya, Peradeniya, Sri Lanka

LESLIE SINN, DVM
Diplomate, American College of Veterinary Behaviorists; Behavior Solutions, Hamilton, Virginia, USA

ELIZABETH STELOW, DVM
Diplomate, American College of Veterinary Behaviorists; Clinical Animal Behavior Service, UC Davis Veterinary Medical Teaching Hospital, Davis, California, USA

BETH GROETZINGER STRICKLER, MS, DVM, CDBC
Diplomate, American College of Veterinary Behaviorists; Veterinary Behavior Solutions, Johnson City, Tennessee, USA

Contents

thorough history will detail each trigger, target, and context and allow for the veterinary team to put together a comprehensive management plan. Management allows for the avoidance of future aggressive episodes and minimizes the risks associated with living with a patient with these diagnoses. Although risk cannot be mitigated 100%, thorough management can create a safe environment for the implementation of the behavior treatment plan.

pets. Treatment of behavior problems in older pets requires a multimodal therapeutic approach. Frequent follow-up visits are required to monitor pets and comment on prognosis. Clients should be informed of the prognosis and should be educated to evaluate pain, discomfort, and general quality of life of the aging pet.

Recent studies have led to some groundbreaking findings regarding the use of medications for the support of behavioral health in dogs and cats. Despite tantalizing results, these studies should be viewed in light of their limitations. Consequently, the results of these studies should be applied in the clinical setting with caution and with a full understanding of the potential pros and cons of using these medications. A review of the research available on trazodone, clonidine, detomidine, dexmedetomidine, propranolol, pindolol, maropitant, memantine, venlafaxine, and gabapentin discusses these pros and cons and highlights key points regarding their clinical use and application.

Behavioral problems of companion animals are becoming more widely recognized. As a result, there are a growing number of behavioral nutraceuticals and diets on the market. These products may be useful for the treatment of mild conditions, for clients who are hesitant to give their pet a psychopharmacologic agent, or sometimes in conjunction with psychopharmacologic agents. Veterinarians should critically review the research associated with nutraceuticals and diets, and have an understanding of the functional ingredients and their mechanisms of action before prescribing treatment. This article provides an overview of nutraceuticals, their mechanisms of action, and relevant research regarding their use.

VETERINARY CLINICS OF NORTH AMERICA: SMALL ANIMAL PRACTICE

THE CLINICS ARE NOW AVAILABLE ONLINE!
Access your subscription at:
www.theclinics.com

Preface

Behavior as Illness Indicator

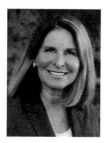

Elizabeth Stelow, DVM
Editor

This issue of *Veterinary Clinics of North America: Small Animal Practice* is the first since May 2014 to focus on behavior problems in cats and dogs. It provides the most current and useful information on both diagnosing and treating common problem behaviors in veterinary patients. As such, it fills a need for both veterinary students and seasoned veterinarians looking for tools to make treating behavior problems a more realistic and manageable endeavor.

The first article, "Diagnosing Behavior Problems: A Guide for Practitioners," focuses on the nuts and bolts of diagnosing problems accurately so that treatment plans are effective. There are aspects of behavior diagnostics that differ substantially from the diagnostic strategies undertaken in medicine cases. For instance, videos of behaviors streamline the process because the clinician can assess the behavior firsthand rather than through the interpretation of the client. The article presents diagnostic criteria for common canine and feline problem behaviors, the ones most likely to be treated by the general practitioner. A section on assessing the prognosis of a behavior case provides useful gauges of the severity of a problem.

Two major dog-specific behavior problems are tackled in "Separation, Confinement, or Noises: What Is Scaring that Dog?" and "Managing Canine Aggression in the Home." In treating canine anxieties, it is crucial to have the correct diagnosis, as treatment plans differ significantly among separation anxiety, confinement anxiety, and noise aversions. This article provides excellent diagnostic criteria and sound treatment options for all three. And, dogs are more likely to present for aggressive behavior, compared to any other behavior problem. The first step in treatment is to manage the dog so that no one is injured and the dog has a break from practicing the undesirable behaviors. Once management strategies are firmly in place, other treatment options, like desensitization and counterconditioning or medication, may be initiated.

The main behavior problem of the cat, inappropriate urination, is discussed in "Vertical or Horizontal: Diagnosing and Treating Cats Who Urinate Outside the Box." As in

Vet Clin Small Anim 48 (2018) ix–x
https://doi.org/10.1016/j.cvsm.2017.12.002
0195-5616/18/© 2017 Published by Elsevier Inc.

other behavior issues, an accurate diagnosis of either urine marking or toileting is crucial to the effectiveness of any treatment plan. This article provides the important diagnostic criteria and treatment options for each of the two problems. Accurate diagnosis and effective treatment of these problems save many cats from relinquishment and euthanasia.

There is perhaps no behavior treatment so seemingly complicated, but actually so straightforward, as desensitization and counterconditioning. The "rules" of keeping the pet under threshold and increasing the strength of the stimulus only gradually are the main predictors of treatment success or failure. Giving the client an accurate description of the goals and principles of, as well as specific strategies for implementing, this behavior modification tool is essential for success. "Desensitization and Counterconditioning: When and How" provides the clinician just that.

Owners of aging pets face many challenges. Older age brings with it the higher likelihood of a pet developing a serious, and potentially life-threatening, medical condition. It also brings the increased pain and the possibility of behavior changes the owners might refer to as "senility." The clinician treating an older pet is more likely to wonder if the behavior changes noted are due to medical problems, primary behavior problems, or a combination. Charting the course of the behavior changes in the older pet can be daunting. "Special Considerations for Diagnosing Behavior Problems in Older Pets" offers concrete guidelines.

The last two articles, "Advances in Behavioral Psychopharmacology" and "Behavioral Nutraceuticals and Diets," explore the possibility of altering brain function as a means to resolving, or perhaps preventing, problem behaviors. A few human medications have recently gained popularity in the treatment of problem behaviors and have been the focus of new research. And several new diets and alternative supplements are now available for everything from anxiety to cognitive dysfunction.

Together, these articles guide the practitioner through a start-to-finish plan for diagnosing and treating common problem behaviors in small animals. I hope they serve their audience well and expand the readers' knowledge of behavioral medicine.

I would like to thank each of the authors for devoting their time to researching and writing about these topics. These authors are among the rising stars of veterinary behavior, each one having completed his or her training and board certification within the past three years. Their future research will, undoubtedly, answer some of the outstanding questions that remain about why pets develop problem behaviors and how best for us to solve them.

Elizabeth Stelow, DVM
UC Davis
Veterinary Medical Teaching Hospital
1 Shields Avenue
Davis, CA 95616, USA

E-mail address:
eastelow@ucdavis.edu

Diagnosing Behavior Problems
A Guide for Practitioners

Elizabeth Stelow, DVM

KEYWORDS

- Canine • Feline • Behavior • Aggression • Anxiety • Behavior history

KEY POINTS

- Clinicians play an important role in diagnosing problem behaviors as a precursor to treating them. This requires a protocol for gathering historical behavioral and health information, direct observation and examination of the animal, and a broad knowledge base of medical and behavioral differential diagnoses for those findings.
- Aggression and anxiety are the most commonly reported behavior problems in dogs. In cats, elimination problems and aggression are the most prevalent. Other important diagnoses for these species are cognitive dysfunction and abnormal repetitive behaviors.
- A diagnosis of aggression should include the target (owners, unfamiliar people, other dogs, other cats, other animals), and the most likely motivation (fear, territoriality, resource guarding, play, and others).
- Fears, phobias, and anxieties require identification of the triggers, whether being left alone, loud noises, or a combination of many triggers, because treatment is directed at the cause.
- The first question to answer in canine and feline elimination problems must be, "Is this urine marking, toileting, or both?" Treatment plans are different for each of these problems.

INTRODUCTION

The role of the veterinary general practitioner in identifying and treating behavior problems among their patients is a crucial one. An estimated 40% of all pet dogs and cats in the United States exhibit problem behaviors.[1,2] These problems take an enormous toll: in numerous studies, behavior problems are listed as the number one reason for relinquishing a dog and the number two reason, behind surrendering entire litters, for relinquishing a cat.[3]

The author has nothing to disclose.
UC Davis, Veterinary Medical Teaching Hospital, 1 Shields Avenue, Davis, CA 95616, USA
E-mail address: eastelow@ucdavis.edu

Vet Clin Small Anim 48 (2018) 339–350
https://doi.org/10.1016/j.cvsm.2017.12.003
0195-5616/18/© 2017 Elsevier Inc. All rights reserved.

Not all veterinarians seem to be equally prepared to address behavioral issues in their patients. In a 2004 article, Siebert and Landsberg[4] outlined findings from several surveys of practicing veterinarians. A 2001 survey by McMillan and Rollin found that only 25% of veterinarians inquire regularly about the patient's behavior.[5] A 2004 survey by Greenfield and colleagues[6] found that veterinarians in small animal practices ranked knowledge about behavior sixteenth among those skills most important for a new veterinary school graduate.

The relative lack of behavior knowledge is apparent to clients, as well. In a 2002 study, Bergman and coworkers[7] found that only 26% of the 500 owners of urine-marking cats that were surveyed had contacted their veterinarians about the problem. The other 74% assumed the veterinarian would be of no help and turned to the Internet and other resources. Of the 70 veterinarians surveyed, only two-thirds could correctly distinguish between urine marking and toileting when given the facts of a case.[7]

One concern is that, in the absence of a good foundation in the diagnosis and treatment of behavioral problems, a clinician's solution might be to send the owners to a nearby trainer to seek resolution. But, thinking of every behavioral problem as a "training problem" and not evaluating the underlying diseases (eg, fear, anxieties), may preclude effective treatment.[8] The two things a veterinarian can do that even the most qualified trainer cannot are to diagnose disease conditions and prescribe medications.

OBSTACLES TO ACCURATE DIAGNOSES
Terminology

One of the more frustrating barriers to a clear, concise behavioral diagnosis is the lack of a consistent, universally accepted lexicon of diagnostic terminology. In many behavioral disorders, the pathophysiologic abnormalities have not been established or agreed on.[8] In others, specialists agree on the basis for certain diagnoses, but not what those diagnoses should be called.[9] The result is that some practitioners use diagnostic categories, whereas others use functional categories to name their diagnoses.[8] Although it would be ideal to have a set naming pattern for behavioral diagnoses, because this would theoretically lead to the most targeted treatment plans, much work has yet to be done.[9] The best a practitioner can do is to be clear in naming a diagnosis about the triggers, response, and context whenever possible.

Confounding Etiologies

Is it medical? Is it behavioral? Is it both? Behavior is often the first noticeable indicator of a medical or disease process; and these processes may affect behavior in several ways:

- An acute illness may present with lethargy, social withdrawal, decreased response to stimuli, decreased appetite, and other signs. It may be that these behaviors are programmed to avoid the spread of disease.[10]
- In chronic disease, behavior changes may be the first clinical signs noted by the owner. Endocrine diseases that cause polyuria and polydipsia may lead to a noticeable increase in water consumption and inappropriate urination. Pain may lead to irritability and reduced activity. Partial seizures may manifest as repetitive behaviors.[10]
- Proinflammatory cytokines, numerous "stress" pathways, gut microbes, medications, dietary supplements, and other factors are increasingly shown to have behavioral manifestations via any number of physiologic processes.[10]

The discussion of medical differentials is presented later.

APPROACH TO DIAGNOSING BEHAVIOR PROBLEMS: AN OVERVIEW

For a practitioner to address problem behaviors among their patients, it is crucial to know what behaviors to screen for. Although the most common problems can change ranking over time, their status in the "top problems" list is consistent.

For dogs, the behavior problems most commonly reported are aggressive behaviors (toward owners, strangers, and other dogs), anxieties (separation, noise, generalized), destructiveness, house-soiling, unruliness, and compulsive behaviors.[2,11] Aggressive behaviors in the dog include growling, snarling, snapping, and biting. In nearly all studies, aggression ranks as the number one unacceptable behavior problem, followed by anxieties.[2,8,11,12]

For cats, the list contains elimination (spraying, toileting), aggression (toward owners, strangers, and other cats), destructiveness, and compulsive behaviors. In most studies, elimination is ranked as the number one behavioral reason for relinquishment of the cat, followed by destructiveness (clawing of furniture) and aggression.[1,8,12,13]

How Is an Accurate Diagnosis Achieved?

When an owner presents a pet for evaluation of a problem behavior, or one is uncovered during a routine vet visit, there are several questions the veterinarian must answer. Is the behavior described or witnessed normal for that species? If so, is there a reason for the owner to find it unacceptable? If not, can I determine why it might have arisen? What medical issues must I rule out to treat the correct underlying cause?[10]

Without further examination, the answers to these questions are usually elusive. Therefore, a complete diagnostic plan should contain the following elements[10]:

- Detailed history (medical and behavioral)
- Observation
- Minimum database
- Knowledge of medical differentials for common problem behaviors
- Understanding of specific diagnostic criteria for common problem behaviors
- Ability to assess prognosis

Each of these is discussed in detail next.

How Can I Get a Detailed History?

A detailed history is the primary diagnostic tool of the behavior case. It is most expedient to use a form that prompts owners for the background details needs. **Table 1** provides recommended elements. Objective descriptions of the behaviors are more useful than subjective assessments of the cause; but, there is often a limit to what the owners can tell you about body language and specific triggers, because most owners do not have a sophisticated awareness of behavior in their pets.[14]

How Can I Best Observe the Problem?

There are two ways of seeing the pet's behavior: direct observation and video provided by the owner. Although in-room observations are important, you may not see the behavior in question. Instead, you will observe how comfortable the pet is in new surroundings and with the owners. You will see whether the owners are nervous about the pet or underestimate the threat it may cause. If two pets are brought for intraspecific fighting, you will see how they interact in a stressful environment; for safety, it is important to have two family members for two dogs, in case tensions rise during the appointment.

Table 1	
Owner history form elements	
Basic information	Signalment and presenting complaint
	Acquisition history (age, source)
	Diet and exercise regimens
	Medical history and current medications/supplements
	Training history, including trainer names, types (private, group, board and train)
Environment	Family members living in the home (humans, other pets)
	Type of home, neighborhood, pet's access in the home and yard
	Whether the pet can see people, cats, or dogs pass by the house; how he reacts when he sees them
Owner description of incidents	What the pet and the owner are doing before, during, and after a typical incident
	Focus on the trigger, the pet's body language and recovery time, and the owner's response to the incident
	The age of onset, progression over time, and current intensity/frequency of the problem
	Number and severity of bites; whether any have been reported to the authorities
	The owner's attempts to correct the problem; outcome of each type of attempt
Owner information	Each owner's level of bond with the pet
	Each owner's goals for outcome

Data from Landsberg G, Hunthausen W, Ackerman L. Behavior problems of the dog and cat. 3rd edition. Edinburgh (United Kingdom): Saunders; 2013.

Before the appointment, ask the owner for video of the pet at home and, if safe to get, an occurrence of a problem. This step is crucial for suspected separation anxiety, because the behaviors occur when no one is home to witness them.[15,16]

How Do I Approach a Physical Examination and Medical Diagnostics?

It is crucial to attempt to identify any influence of medical issues on behavior. Changes in behavior are the first signs of emerging medical problems. There is a higher index of suspicion of an underlying medical condition when the behavior change is sudden or appears later in life.[17,18] Most behavior issues in the dog arise at a mean age of 2.5 years (except anxieties, at an average 6.5 years).[2] In cats, the mean age for presentation of behavior problems is 5.5 years (except ingestive problems at closer to 1.5 years).[13] Thus, if a middle-aged dog suddenly becomes aggressive or anxious, extra care should be spent on medical diagnostics and physical examination.

Beyond a physical examination, a thorough work-up includes basic laboratory work (complete blood count, serum biochemistry panel, urinalysis, T4 in the cat), and any other laboratory test warranted by physical examination findings. For possible joint pain or uroliths, consider radiographs. Gastrointestinal differentials may require ultrasound or endoscopy.[10,18]

DIAGNOSTIC CRITERIA FOR SPECIFIC PROBLEMS
Aggression

Aggression, particularly toward people, is the number one diagnosed behavior problem in dogs and the number two in cats.[1,13,19] Therefore, it is important for the general practitioner to be able to diagnose and treat it effectively.

One challenge is that "aggression" is not a complete behavioral diagnosis; rather, it is a clinical sign of a medical or behavioral problem.[20] Perhaps for that reason, aggression is an easy and a difficult diagnosis to make. We all think we know it when we see (or read owner accounts about) it. Yet, sometimes a clinician is uncertain about the true nature of the behavior described. Video can aid the diagnosis, based on the behavior and body language of the patient.

Once aggressive behaviors have been identified, the actual diagnosis requires defining the motivation behind them and the victims. Possible victims include owners, strangers, or both; other dogs inside and outside the household; other cats in the household; or other species.[11,13]

The part of the diagnosis that involves motivation is often more complicated. Considering just two published sources, one can see the wide variety of motivations attributed to canine aggression: maternal (toward people or pups), redirected, food-related, possessive, predatory, impulse-control, idiopathic, conflict-related, resource guarding, fear-related, territorial/protective, pain-induced/irritable, play, dominance-related, intraspecific miscommunication, intraspecific dominance/status-related, and pathophysiologic.[9,10] Many of these represent different flavors of "fear," including territorial, redirected, food/resource guarding, possessive, and pain-related. Also, "dominance" aggression can apply only to intraspecific aggression and does not include aggression toward people.[21]

Feline aggression is often divided into the following categories: play/predatory, fear-related, petting-induced, redirected, pain-induced, territorial, intercat (household), and hormonally mediated. Play aggression sounds harmless but can inflict sometimes-severe injury on people; it is characterized by stalking before an attack. Petting-induced aggression may happen after a few pets or several minutes of petting.[10]

To determine which motivations are most likely in a given case, the context and the body language of the animal are both relevant. Unfortunately, owners are not equally skilled at providing this information. Unless the aggression occurs in the presence of the clinician, there is sometimes incomplete information about motivation, which is important mainly because of its effect on prognosis.[10]

Inappropriate Elimination

Although cats and dogs sometimes relieve themselves in the house, they often have different reasons for doing so. For the problem to be properly addressed, diagnostics must uncover the reason.[9]

Feline elimination
For cats, inappropriate elimination is the number one reported problem behavior.[9] It can take two main forms: toileting/litter box aversion and urine marking. It is essential that the clinician distinguish between these early in the diagnostic process, because the treatments are different.[7] The article by Leticia Mattos de Souza Dantas', article "Vertical or Horizontal? Diagnosing and Treating Cats Who Urinate Outside the Box," in this issue provides a thorough differentiation between feline urine marking and toileting.

Feline toileting Inappropriate toileting in cats results when a cat voids the contents of its bladder or rectum someplace other than the litter box. With inappropriate urination, in contrast to urine marking, the urine is most often left on a horizontal surface and the cat is often seen in a typical squatting posture of urination. Cats may even dig before or after inappropriate toileting.[22]

The cat may be avoiding the litter box for any of several reasons. Commonly, there is recent history of a lower urinary tract or constipation problem that caused pain in the litter box. The cat does not want to risk that pain again, so chooses a different substrate or location. As his issue resolves and urination/defecation no longer hurts, he finds that this new substrate is more comfortable than the litter box.

Other reasons include a new box/litter/location that the cat does not like, poor litter box hygiene, another cat creating social tension near the box, mobility problems that make getting to or into the box difficult, or something scary happening near the box. A good history and medical diagnostics often uncover everything necessary for this diagnosis. If either urine or feces are left in the box (but not the other) chances are there is an underlying medical problem versus a problem with the box.[10,22]

Feline urine marking Urine marking has little to do with the litter box. In fact, most marking cats still urinate and defecate in their box. Urine marking is a chemical signal to other cats. If owners witness the marking behavior, they generally note a small amount of urine being deposited on a socially significant vertical surface (eg, threshold, bannister) by a cat that is treading with his back feet while his tail quivers and he stares with eyes half closed into the distance.[22] It is less common for small amounts of urine or feces to be left on socially significant horizontal surfaces; and most horizontally marking cats also mark vertical surfaces.[10,22]

Urine marking, as a form of communication, is a normal behavior outdoors, but unacceptable indoors. It is most often attributable to the presence of outdoor cats around the house; challenging social dynamics among indoor cats; or changes within the home or family, including moves, new people/pets, and schedule changes. An adequate history, along with the reports of small amounts of urine on vertical surfaces, are typically enough to make a tentative diagnosis.[10]

The medical differentials for urine marking and urination include urinary tract infection, calculi, neoplasia, hyperthyroid, feline interstitial cystitis, feline leukemia virus, and feline immunodeficiency virus. For defecation outside the box, differentials include tenesmus, dyschezia, and feline infectious peritonitis.[18]

Canine elimination

The dog that urinates or defecates in the home may also do so for a variety of reasons. Urination can be toileting or urine marking, just as in cats. Toileting, if behavioral in nature, is most likely attributable to either incomplete house training or inadequate access to the outdoors to eliminate. If lapses in house training happen only when the owners are gone, separation anxiety or other cause of autonomic stimulation should be explored. Submissive and excitement urination happen at specific times and in the presence of people, so are easy to identify. Medical differentials to consider include urinary or gastrointestinal inflammatory processes, any cause of polyuria/polydipsia or diarrhea, or cognitive decline.[9]

Urine marking in the home is far less common in dogs than cats. It may reflect social tension among household dogs, concern over dogs that pass by windows, undesired visitors to the home, or other cause of stress or trigger of territoriality. The biggest challenge with the diagnosis of urine marking in the dog is that the posture assumed is usually identical to that of toileting.[9,10]

Anxieties, Fears, and Phobias

Both colloquially and in veterinary literature, there is great overlap and confusion among the terms "fear," "phobia," and "anxiety." For the purpose of this discussion, anxiety is a state of arousal as a response to uncertainty or the prospect of real or imagined danger. Its clinical signs are fairly nonspecific and include increased respiratory and heart rate, trembling, increased salivation, pacing, circling, seeking closeness, and transient anorexia.[23,24]

A phobia is an excessive and usually persistent fear of a specific and discernible object or situation. Responses include autonomic arousal and marked behavior signs, often directed at escape.[23,24]

Fear represents sympathetic alarm response to a threatened or present danger. It occurs most often in proximity to the threatening stimulus and is typically brief in duration. Specific fear behaviors fall into several categories, including classic fear responses (panting, shaking, trembling, pacing, whining), avoidance behaviors (escape attempts, hiding, destructiveness, digging, frantic running), and attention-seeking (pawing at or following owner).[18,25] Unlike anxieties and phobias, fear, in response to a legitimate threat, is an adaptive response.[23,24,26]

There are several categories of fear that require different types of treatment. Simple fears are those that are triggered by a single, identifiable stimulus. Complex fears are those with multiple triggering stimuli that cause increased anxiety between triggers. Phobias, as described previously, are extreme responses and can include panic. A good history of the problem can distinguish among these fear types. The development of fearful behaviors seems to vary by type. Some fears seem to be associated with a traumatic exposure. Others seem to be a function of lack of exposure during a formative period or sensitization via repeated exposure. Genetics is a risk factor, as is social transmission via exposure to another animal expressing fear.[23,27]

In general, the fear/anxiety/phobia behavior issues we most commonly diagnose and treat as veterinarians include separation anxiety, noise aversions, and generalized anxiety disorder. Separation, confinement, and noise aversions are discussed in detail in Kelly C. Ballantyne's article, "Separation, Confinement, or Noises: What Is Scaring that Dog?," in this issue. Generalized anxiety has a different presentation than the others and is discussed later.

Separation Anxiety

Separation anxiety is defined as "problematic behavior associated with anxiety that occurs exclusively in the owner's absence or virtual absence".[16] Canine separation anxiety is thought to affect between 14% and 17% of dogs in the United States and 20% in the United Kingdom.[24] It is a challenge for owners and makes the dog a higher risk for relinquishment because of the stress it places on the owner's relationship with the pet.[24]

Feline separation anxiety has been studied far less than the canine variety, perhaps because of the relative infrequency with which it is reported. Because of the paucity of research on the subject, conjectures about prevalence in the feline population have not been made. Clinical signs most commonly reported are inappropriate elimination (with urination most commonly on the owner's bed), excessive vocalization, destructiveness, and overgrooming.[28]

The clinical signs of canine separation anxiety

A dog that is left alone may exhibit one or many nonspecific signs of anxiety. Most commonly reported are destruction, urination/defecation, self-harm, and/or vocalization; these are reported because the owner can see tangible signs of them or hear reports from neighbors.[29] Other, less obvious signs of anxiety that may occur include panting, freezing, drooling, trembling, restlessness, transient anorexia, and withdrawal. These more subtle signs are noted only with video recording during the time of the owner absence.[15]

Differential diagnoses

There are several medical and behavioral differentials that should be considered for separation anxiety. Destructiveness or rearranging household items can represent hepatic encephalopathy, other anxieties, or cognitive decline. Urination or defecation can signal cystitis, causes of polyuria/polydipsia, seizures, gastrointestinal disease, or high dietary fiber. They may also result from being left without access to an elimination area or being incompletely housetrained. Excessive salivation can be caused by toxin exposure or nausea. Distress vocalization may indicate hepatic encephalopathy, aggression, noise aversion/panic, or social facilitation with a nearby dog. Finally, self-trauma may suggest allergies, neuritis, hepatic encephalopathy, parasites, or a displacement or compulsive repetitive behavior.[24,30]

Noise Aversions

Another pervasive anxiety, in dogs in particular, is noise aversions. The most common noises reported to create fear include thunder, fireworks, gunshots, and any other type of explosion.[24,25,27,31] Its prevalence in the canine population is between 20% and 50%.[23,24,31]

Diagnosis is based entirely on a history of the dog reacting to specific types of noises with any of the fear behaviors described previously.[31] It is important to note from the history how quickly the animal recovers from a fearful incident and whether there is anxiety between incidents, because this can greatly influence the treatment plan.[27] If the types of noises are widely varied and the dog has other types of triggers, the practitioner should consider that a more complex fear or phobia is at play.

Reported differential diagnoses are sparse, but include cognitive dysfunction and hypothyroid (dogs).[23]

Generalized Anxiety

Generalized anxiety is described as a persistent condition reflecting autonomic hyperactivity, hyperreactivity, and hypervigilance, interfering with normal daily social and maintenance behaviors.[9] The dogs are noted by owners to be surveying their surroundings constantly, and usually unable to focus when even slightly "outside their comfort zone."[9] They exhibit an extreme or out-of-context reaction to stimuli that includes panting, pacing, and/or lunging at triggers; in fact, aggression may be the actual presenting complaint. There may be a persistent diarrhea.[9]

Differentials diagnoses

Medical differentials include pain, endocrinopathies, and cardiac disease. In older dogs, cognitive decline should be considered. If the dog has diarrhea, rule out inflammatory bowel diseases, as necessary.[9]

Abnormal Repetitive Behaviors

Abnormal (sometimes called "maladaptive") repetitive behaviors in dogs and cats are a varied and poorly defined group of diagnoses, the causes of which are not well understood. Included among these diagnoses are stereotypic, compulsive, and displacement behaviors. The predisposing factors are shared among them and include genetics, conflict, frustration, and anxiety.[32]

Stereotypic behaviors

Stereotypies are patterned and unvarying and serve no clear purpose. Examples include carnivores pacing in zoos and cribbing horses. The key types of stereotypy are oral (hooved stock and primates) and locomotor (carnivores and rodents). The specific predisposing factor seems to be frustration, often caused by extreme confinement. For that reason, few cats and dogs are diagnosed with stereotypic behaviors. One rare exception is a kenneled dog that develops a repetitive locomotor behavior.[33]

Compulsive behaviors

These are far more common than stereotypes in cats and dogs. They are locomotor (tail chasing, spinning), hallucinatory (fly-snapping), self-injurious (acral lick), and oral (pica, flank sucking). Two hallmarks of compulsive behaviors are that they are not easily interrupted and they tend to interfere with normal maintenance activities.[32,34] The typical age of onset of compulsive behaviors is 12 to 36 months for dogs and 24 to 48 months for cats. Many of the cats and dogs diagnosed with compulsive behaviors have one or more concurrent behavior diagnoses, including aggression, separation anxiety, attention seeking, and others.[34] Medical differentials for compulsive behaviors include primary gastrointestinal disease, pain, pruritus, seizure activity, and urinary tract disease.[32,35]

Displacement behaviors

The third category of repetitive behaviors is displacement behaviors, which are any normal behavior that is displayed out of context as a response to conflict between two competing motivations; the chosen behavior seems irrelevant in the setting it is produced. An example is a dog that wishes to eat but whose dish is guarded by an aggressive conspecific; in this context, the dog chooses to groom himself, displaying what can only be perceived as a displacement behavior.[36]

Cognitive Dysfunction

The aging brain is prone to several changes that, although anatomic or physiologic in nature, affect behavior. These include the buildup of β-amyloid plaques in the hippocampus and cerebral cortex; reduced glucose uptake and metabolism in the brain; oxidative damage in the brain; and perivascular changes, including arteriosclerosis and infarcts. What the owner notices is commonly thought of as cognitive decline.[10]

The clinical signs of cognitive dysfunction in the dog are disorientation, changes in social interactions, loss of housetraining, disturbances in the sleep-wake cycle, and changes in activity levels or ability to learn. Medical differentials include thyroid abnormalities, diabetes, pain, seizure activities, and other diffuse brain or central nervous system disease.[10]

In the cat, the most common clinical signs are increased vocalization, nighttime restlessness, loss of housetraining, disorientation, aggression, and anxiety. Medical differentials include pain, thyroid disease, renal disease, hypertension, and forebrain disease.[4]

For a more complete discussion on cognitive dysfunction, see Eranda Rajapaksha's article, "Special Considerations for Diagnosing Behavior Problems in Older Pets," in this issue.

ASSESSING PROGNOSIS

A behavior evaluation is not complete without offering the owner an assessment of prognosis. **Table 2** shows all the elements to be considered before formulating a prognosis.

Each plan likely has management elements that avoid allowing the pet to practice its unwanted behaviors; prognosis relies heavily on the owners' acceptance of and ability to implement these management strategies. Other key factors include age of onset and duration of the problem, predictability, and response to treatment.[9] It is important to assess how the client reacts to finding that the goal of treatment of most behavior

Table 2
Elements of a behavioral prognosis

Pet factors	How well-diagnosed is the problem?
	Is the pet otherwise healthy?
	How severe are the clinical signs?
	How recently did the pet develop this behavior?
	How predictable is the behavior?
	How easily can the stimuli be controlled or removed?
	How high is the risk of injury?
Owner factors	How interested are the clients in understanding the diagnoses?
	How committed are the owners to the pet?
	How much work is this pet for these owners?
	How familiar are the owners with behavior modification techniques?
	Can these owners refrain from punishing their pet?
	How capable are the owners of implementing the plan?
	How reasonable are the owners' goals?

Data from Overall KL. Manual of clinical behavioral medicine for dogs and cats. St Louis (MO): Mosby; 2013; and Landsberg G, Hunthausen W, Ackerman L. Behavior problems of the dog and cat. 3rd edition. Edinburgh (United Kingdom): Saunders; 2013.

problems is to control, not to cure, and that response to treatment is more unpredictable than most medical conditions.[8] Still, client compliance is likely the single most important factor in prognosis.[9]

SUMMARY

The remainder of this issue, full of articles written by the fresh voices of veterinary behavior, lays out the treatment plans recommended for the behavior problems described previously. Together, they work as a complete game plan for some of the key behavior problems a clinician is likely to diagnose.

REFERENCES

1. Amat M, Ruiz de la Torre JL, Fatjó J, et al. Potential risk factors associated with feline behavior problems. Appl Anim Behav Sci 2009;121:134–9.
2. Martinez AG, Pernas GS, Casalta FJD, et al. Risk factors associated with behavioral problems in dogs. J Vet Behav 2011;6:225–31.
3. Salman MD, Hutchison JM, Ruch-Gallie R, et al. Behavioral reasons for relinquishment of dogs and cats to 12 shelters. J Appl Anim Welf Sci 2000;3:93–106.
4. Seibert LM, Landsberg GM. Diagnosis and management of patients presenting with behavior problems. Vet Clin North Am Small Anim Pract 2008;38:937–50.
5. McMillan FD, Rollin BE. The presence of mind: on reunifying the animal mind and body. J Am Vet Med Assoc 2001;218(11):1723–7.
6. Greenfield CL, Johnson AL, Schaeffer DJ. Frequency of use of various procedures, skills, and areas of knowledge among veterinarians in private small animal exclusive or predominant practice and proficiency expected of new veterinary school graduates. J Am Vet Med Assoc 2004;224(11):1780–7.
7. Bergman L, Hart BL, Bain M, et al. Evaluation of urine marking by cats as a model for understanding veterinary diagnostic and treatment approaches and client attitudes. J Am Vet Med Assoc 2002;221:1282–6.
8. Horwitz DF. Differences and similarities between behavioral and internal medicine. J Am Vet Med Assoc 2000;217:1372–6.

9. Overall KL. Manual of clinical behavioral medicine for dogs and cats. St Louis (MO): Mosby; 2013.
10. Landsberg G, Hunthausen W, Ackerman L. Behavior problems of the dog and cat. 3rd edition. Edinburgh (United Kingdom): Saunders; 2013.
11. Bamberger M, Houpt KA. Signalment factors, comorbidity, and trends in behavior diagnoses in dogs: 1644 cases (1991–2001). J Am Vet Med Assoc 2006;229: 1591–601.
12. Podberscek AL. Positive and negative aspects of our relationship with companion animals. Vet Res Commun 2006;30:21–7.
13. Bamberger M, Houpt KA. Signalment factors, comorbidity, and trends in behavior diagnoses in cats: 736 cases (1991-2001). J Am Vet Med Assoc 2006;229: 1602–6.
14. Mariti C, Gazzano A, Moore JL, et al. Perception of dogs' stress by their owners. J Vet Behav 2012;7:213–9.
15. Palestrini C, Minero M, Cannas S, et al. Video analysis of dogs with separation-related behaviors. Appl Anim Behav Sci 2010;124:61–7.
16. Cannas S, Frank D, Minero M, et al. Video analysis of dogs suffering from anxiety when left home alone and treated with clomipramine. J Vet Behav 2014;9:50–7.
17. Overall KL. Medical differentials with potential behavioral manifestations. Vet Clin North Am Small Anim Pract 2003;33:213–29.
18. Frank D. Recognizing behavioral signs of pain and disease: a guide for practitioners. Vet Clin North Am Small Anim Pract 2014;44:507–24.
19. Fatjó J, Amat M, Mariotti VM, et al. Analysis of 1040 cases of canine aggression in a referral practice in Spain. J Vet Behav 2007;2:158–65.
20. Sueda KLC, Malamed R. Canine aggression toward people: a guide for the practitioner. Vet Clin North Am Small Anim Pract 2014;44:599–628.
21. Yin S. Low stress handling, restraint and behavior modification of dogs and cats. Davis (CA): CattleDog Publishing; 2009. p. 52–73.
22. Rodan I, Heath S. Feline behavioral health and welfare prevention and treatment. St Louis (MO): Elsevier; 2016.
23. Mills D. Management of noise fears and phobias in pets. Practice 2005;27: 248–55.
24. Sherman BL, Mills DS. Canine anxieties and phobias: an update on separation anxiety and noise aversions. Vet Clin North Am Small Anim Pract 2008;38: 1081–106.
25. McCobb EC, Brown EA, Damiani K, et al. Thunderstorm phobia in dogs: an Internet survey of 69 cases. J Am Anim Hosp Assoc 2001;37:319–24.
26. Tiira K, Sulkama S, Lohi H. Prevalence, co-morbidity and behavioral variation in canine anxiety. J Vet Behav 2016;16:36–44.
27. Levine ED. Sound sensitivities. In: Horwitz D, Mills D, editors. BSAVA manual of canine and feline behavioural medicine. Quedgeley (United Kingdom): British Small Animal Veterinary Association; 2009. p. 159–68.
28. Schwartz S. Separation anxiety syndrome in dogs and cats. J Am Vet Med Assoc 2003;222:1526–32.
29. Storengen LM, Boge SCK, Strøm SJ, et al. A descriptive study of 215 dogs diagnosed with separation anxiety. Appl Anim Behav Sci 2014;159:82–9.
30. Voith VL, Borchelt PL. Separation anxiety in dogs. Compend Contin Educ Pract Vet 1985;7(1):42–52.
31. Blackwell EJ, Bradshaw JWS, Casey RA. Fear responses to noises in domestic dogs: prevalence, risk factors and co-occurrence with other fear related behaviour. Appl Anim Behav Sci 2013;145:15–25.

32. Tynes VV, Sinn L. Abnormal repetitive behaviors in cats and dogs: a guide for practitioners. Vet Clin North Am Small Anim Pract 2014;44:543–64.

33. Rushen J, Mason G. A decade-or-more's progress in understanding stereotypic behavior. In: Mason G, Rushen J, editors. Stereotypic animal behaviour: fundamentals and applications to welfare. 2nd edition. Wallingford (WA): CABI; 2006. p. 1–18.

34. Overall KL, Dunham AE. Clinical features and outcome in dogs and cats with obsessive–compulsive disorder: 126 cases (1989-2000). J Am Vet Med Assoc 2002;221:1445–52.

35. Zulch HE, Mills DE, Lambert R, et al. The use of tramadol in a Labrador Retriever presented with self-mutilation of the tail. J Vet Behav 2012;7:252–8.

36. Hetts S, Heinke ML, Estep DQ. Behavior wellness concepts for general veterinary practice. J Am Vet Med Assoc 2004;225:506–13.

FURTHER READINGS

Flannigan G, Dodman NH. Risk factors and behaviors associated with separation anxiety in dogs. J Am Vet Med Assoc 2001;219:460–6.

Overall KL, Dunham AE, Frank D. Frequency of nonspecific clinical signs in dogs with separation anxiety, thunderstorm phobia, and noise phobia, alone or in combination. J Am Vet Med Assoc 2001;219:467–73.

Patronek GJ, Glickman LT, Beck AM, et al. Risk factors for the relinquishment of dogs to an animal shelter. J Am Vet Med Assoc 1996;209:572–81.

Perry G, Seksel K, Beer L, et al. Separation anxiety: a summary of some of the characteristics of 61 cases seen at a Sydney, Australia behaviour practice. In: Mills D, Levine E, Landsberg G, et al, editors. Current issues and research in veterinary behavioral medicine. West Lafayette (IN): Purdue University Press; 2005. p. 280–2.

Scarlett JM, Salman MD, New JG, et al. The role of veterinary practitioners in reducing dog and cat relinquishments and euthanasias. J Am Vet Med Assoc 2002;220:306–11.

Voith VL. The impact of companion animal problems on society and the role of veterinarians. Vet Clin North Am Small Anim Pract 2009;39:327–45.

Wright JC, Nesselrote MS. Classification of behavior problems in dogs: distributions of age, breed, sex and reproductive status. Appl Anim Behav Sci 1987;19:169–78.

Developing a Plan to Treat Behavior Disorders

Isabelle Demontigny-Bédard, DMV, MSc[a],*, Diane Frank, DMV[b]

KEYWORDS

- Behavioral disorders • Management • Training tools • Psychotropic medication

KEY POINTS

- Veterinarians must collect a complete history of the behavioral complaint as well as presence of any other signs (eg, dermatologic or gastrointestinal signs).
- Management (avoiding triggers, predictable interactions, safe areas, choices for the animal, etc) can be implemented immediately.
- Coercive training methods are controversial and there is no evidence that aversive training techniques are more effective than reward-based training techniques.
- Dog training should therefore rely on positive reinforcement methods and avoid positive punishment and negative reinforcement as much as possible.
- Psychotropic medication is prescribed to animals with a behavioral disorder (abnormal behavior), showing signs of anxiety, and/or increased reactivity.

INTRODUCTION

Developing a plan to treat behavior disorders has been broken down into 4 general steps. The first 2 are services easily offered by all veterinarians (ie, complete history and management). Training methods, particularly aversive techniques, are controversial, and can result in physical injuries and emotional consequences (fear and anxiety). Behavior modification based on positive reinforcement (rewards) is, thus, highly recommended. Choice of medication and pharmacologic follow-up will depend on signs of the behavioral disorder, including anxiety and reactivity.

Disclosure Statement: The authors have nothing to disclose.
[a] Centre Vétérinaire DMV, Centre DMV, 2300, 54th Avenue, Montreal, Québec H8T 3R2, Canada;
[b] Department of Clinical Sciences, Faculty of Veterinary Medicine, University of Montreal, 3200 Sicotte, Saint-Hyacinthe, Québec J2S 7C6, Canada
* Corresponding author.
E-mail address: isabelledemontigny@gmail.com

HISTORY OF BEHAVIORAL COMPLAINTS AND OTHER SIGNS
Undesirable Versus Abnormal Behaviors

Behavior can be normal but undesirable or abnormal. Five criteria can be used to make this distinction:

1. Context: Is the behavior appropriate for the context?
2. Behavioral sequence: Is there an alteration of the behavioral sequence?
3. Frequency: Is the frequency appropriate for the context?
4. Severity or duration: Is the severity (or duration) of the behavior justified for the context?
5. Occurrence of anxiety-related behaviors: Does the animal exhibit anxiety-related behaviors in one or multiple contexts?

Undesirable normal behaviors can usually be managed with appropriate training methods. Training alone will most probably not be enough to address abnormal behaviors efficiently and humanely. Abnormal behaviors (medical and behavioral disorders) are characterized by one or several of the following: the behavior is inappropriate for the context, the behavior sequence is modified, or the frequency, the severity or the duration are excessive or unjustified for the context.

Behavioral, Medical, or Both?

In the case of abnormal behavior, the veterinarian must assess the patient and diagnose if the changes result from a medical or a behavioral disorder (**Fig. 1**). Medical conditions, painful or not, can trigger abnormal behaviors. For example, a dog in pain can be more prone to exhibit aggression when approached or touched.[1] A cat with renal insufficiency urinates greater amounts and, if the litter box is not cleaned accordingly, it can lead to house soiling.[2] Therefore, a thorough medical history should be obtained for all patients presented with a behavioral complaint. Physical examination, a complete blood cell count, serum chemistry, total thyroxine measurement, and urinalysis may all be warranted.

As scientific knowledge increases, some signs that have long been considered to stem from behavioral disorders may be found to have a medical component. For example, compulsive disorders are characterized by abnormal and repetitive behaviors that may vary and are oriented toward a goal.[3] They arise in a situation of conflict or frustration and emancipate from this context.[3] This diagnosis is made when all possible medical causes are ruled out.[3] Recent studies have identified gastrointestinal disorders in dogs presented with excessive licking of surfaces, fly biting, and star gazing, which have frequently been diagnosed as compulsive behaviors.[4-6]

Gut–Brain Axis

The bidirectional communication between the brain and the gastrointestinal system has been recognized and is now being studied. The gut–brain axis is composed of the central nervous system, neuroendocrine system, neuroimmune system, the sympathetic and parasympathetic branches of the autonomic nervous system, the enteric nervous system and the intestinal microbiota.[7,8] These components interact mainly via inflammatory mediators, neurotransmitters, hormones, and metabolites.[9]

More than 90% of the body's serotonin is produced in the intestine by enterochromaffin cells.[10] Serotonin blood levels are lower in germ-free mice.[9] Germ-free rats and mice also experience an increased release of adrenocorticotrophic hormone and corticosterone, resulting in a dysregulation of the hypothalamic–pituitary–adrenal axis.[7-9,11]

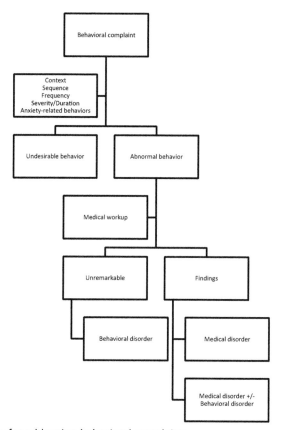

Fig. 1. Algorithm for addressing behavioral complaints.

These findings highlight the importance of the gut microbiota in the normal functioning of the gut–brain axis and stress response. They can also shed light on why some conditions that were thought to be strictly behavioral may also have a gastrointestinal component. It is, therefore, crucial to collect all the clinical signs in any given patient to address the various systems involved.

Stress, Anxiety, and Dermatologic Conditions

As with the gut–brain axis, an interplay between the brain and skin exists. Self-induced alopecia unrelated to a medical cause is compatible with psychogenic alopecia.[12] It is a diagnosis of exclusion.[13] In 1 study of 21 cats with a presumptive diagnosis of psychogenic alopecia, 16 cats (76%) had a medical cause of pruritus.[14] Three cats (14%) had a medical cause of pruritus and psychogenic alopecia.[14] Only 2 cats (10%) were ultimately diagnosed with psychogenic alopecia alone.[14] Skin scrapings, fungal culture, parasiticides, exclusion diet, assessment for atopy, and endocrinopathies and skin biopsies were done on each cat.[14]

In humans, there is a link between stress and increased epidermal permeability.[15] A study on hairless mice suggested that the increased production of glucocorticoids secondary to psychological stress is responsible for altering the permeability barrier homeostasis.[16] Therefore, atopic diseases could potentially be exacerbated by stress in predisposed animals.[17] Interestingly, in 1 study of 21 dogs with recurrent pyoderma, psychogenic factors were identified in 47.6% of cases and 33.3% were improved with behavioral treatment.[18] And, in a retrospective survey-based study, dogs with extreme nonsocial fear and separation anxiety had an increased severity and frequency of skin disorders.[19]

The relation between stress and anxiety and dermatologic conditions or between stress and anxiety and digestive conditions emphasizes the importance of treating both the medical and behavioral components when present concurrently.

MANAGEMENT

Management is essential in the treatment of behavior disorders. If well-implemented, management techniques can prevent worsening of the problem. Specific management options vary depending on the problematic behavior. However, some general principles apply.

Avoid Triggers

First, triggers for the problematic behavior should be identified when possible. Then, every effort should be made initially to avoid or decrease their intensity or frequency (**Table 1**). As the old saying states, "practice makes perfect." Every time an animal has the opportunity to exhibit a behavior, the better he or she becomes at doing so. The animal learns and physiologic changes occur in the brain. When neurons are fired together, there is an increase in strength of the interneural connections.[20] Therefore, the response is more likely to happen in the future in a similar situation.

Predictable Interactions

Many behavioral disorders stem from or are linked to anxiety. Increasing consistency and predictability during daily interactions between owners and pets can help to decrease anxiety or stress. Several names have been given to protocols that implement predictable interactions and improve communication between owner and dog. "Nothing in life is free," "Doggy please," "Protocol for deference," and "Learn to earn" are a few examples.[21–24] These protocols have the dog perform a simple and calm behavior that he or she knows such as "sit" before any interaction with the owner. Therefore, the dog learns a desirable behavior to obtain consequences he or she wants or needs. If the consequences are always neutral or positive, he or she also learns that the owner is a reliable source of information. Sit means nothing bad will happen. Cats can also be taught to sit before interactions.

Table 1
Problematic behaviors with possible avoidance strategies

Problematic Behavior	Avoidance Strategy
Aggression toward visitors	Confinement when visitors are expected
Barking at windows	Block access, cover windows
Destruction when left alone	Boarding, daycare, dog or cat sitter, bring to work
Fighting between animals within the household	Separate when not supervised
Food aggression	Confinement when eating
Leash reactivity	Avoid walks, walk at low-traffic times, walk in low-traffic areas, walk when few dogs or people are around, and so on

Provide Safe and Quiet Spots

Cats and dogs should have a secure and calm place when they want or need to retreat or get away from triggers. They should be able to recognize this location as their own (ie, no one will disturb them when they are in that area). This safe place can be anywhere in the home but needs to always be easily accessible.

Examples of safe refuges for dogs
- Crate
- Dog bed or mat in a quiet room

Examples of safe refuges for cats
- Carrier
- Room with water, food, bedding, and scratching post
- Cupboard (door always left partially open) with bedding
- Cat tree or shelves

Understanding Body Language

Owners able to recognize signs of canine or feline fear, anxiety, or stress (**Table 2**) will be able to act promptly in a situation in which their pet feels uncomfortable. They may choose to remove their dog or cat as calmly as possible from the situation and, thus, may prevent aggravation of the problem.

Safe Interactions Between Children and Dogs

The complex issue of dog bites stems largely from the lack of accurate data. Not all bites are reported. The severity of bites varies greatly from case to case. Breed identification is subjective and often inaccurate.[25,26] Some aggression is "abnormal" and some aggression is appropriate ("self-defense" against a threat or danger), yet no distinction is made based on context or severity of the injuries.

One study showed that most dog bites to younger children occurred indoors, with familiar dogs, during positive interactions initiated by the child.[27] Another study revealed that food guarding was the most common circumstance for bites to familiar children.[28] One survey of 804 dog owners revealed that there is a general lack of

Table 2
Signs of fear, anxiety, or stress

	Cat	Dog
Ears	Flat to the side or back	Back
Eyes	Dilated pupils	Droopy Avoiding gaze
Mouth	Lip licking repeatedly	Lip licking Panting Yawning repeatedly
Tail	Flicking	Down or tucked under the body
Hair	Piloerection	Piloerection
Body posture	Low or tensed, crouching	Low or tensed
Behavior	Hissing Hiding	Increased vigilance Pacing Moving away Refusing treats Growling

knowledge about dog aggression toward children.[29] Another study of dog bites to children (n = 100) stated that the vast majority of bites occurred in the absence of adult supervision and two-thirds of the bites could have been prevented with proper education of parents and children.[30] Adult supervision of child–dog interactions is, therefore, essential with any dog.

Education on safe interactions between children and dogs is also essential.[31]

- Do not approach a dog while he or she is eating.
- Do not disturb a dog while he or she is sleeping or lying down.
- Do not hug or kiss the dog.
- Interact gently with the dog: do not scream at the dog, hit the dog, pull on the dog's ears, tail, or fur, or climb on the dog.
- Ask for owner permission to approach and/or touch the dog. Approach slowly, pat the dog under the chin or on the chest, avoid direct eye contact, and walk away slowly.
- Do not approach a dog without an owner present (tied outdoors, in a car, etc).

Sterilization

Some positives changes in problematic behaviors can be seen with sterilization. A significant reduction or resolution of urine marking in approximately 90% of adult male cats occurs after castration.[32] Only 10% of castrated male and 5% of spayed females exhibit urine marking.[33]

Castration of adult male dogs decreased roaming in 90%, fighting with other males in 60%, mounting of other dogs or people in 60%, and urine marking in 50% of cases.[34] Castration of adult male dogs improved urine marking, mounting, and roaming by at least 50% in at least 60% of dogs and by at least 90% in 25% to 40% of dogs.[35] Castration had no significant effect on fear of inanimate stimuli and aggression toward unfamiliar people.[35] Therefore, neutering should be considered to treat urine marking, roaming, aggression between male dogs, and mounting. Neutering, even if it does not generally result in reduced aggression, is also recommended for any intact aggressive animal because this individual may not be suitable for breeding.[36]

Choice: Environmental Enrichment

Environmental enrichment for confined animals has been studied in laboratory settings, zoos, and shelter situations. The goal of enrichment is to decrease the impact of external stressors and increase the well-being and quality of life of the animal. Examples of environmental enrichment for cats typically include supplying a variety of toys, availability of food and presentation (food distributors, puzzle feeders, hiding the food in variable locations, offering a choice for the type of food), as well as offering opportunities to climb (cat trees, shelves), scratch, and hide.[37,38] The hiding places should have safe entries and exits. In multicat households, several feeding and elimination areas should be available to increase privacy[39] and decrease potential aggressive interactions between cats that tolerate each other from a distance. Sensory enrichment can include provision of catnip or cat grass, or access to an outdoor enclosure. Other options of enrichment consist of social interactions with the cat such as actively playing, combing, brushing, petting, or teaching new behaviors. Individuals will vary in their preferences so it may involve some trial and error to find out what a given cat actually prefers.

One study investigated 3 environmental enrichment choices for 26 shelter cats.[40] Cats could choose to stay in an empty control compartment, a compartment with a prey-simulating toy, a compartment with a perching opportunity, or a compartment with a hiding opportunity. These cats spent a significantly greater percentage of time in the hiding compartment compared with the toy or control compartments. Anecdotally, even in a familiar home setting, some cats may hide to rest. Hiding places can range from cardboard boxes and tents to higher locations where the cat is "unreachable" or "invisible." Providing hiding places gives the cat options that he or she may or may not choose.

More attention to reduce stress within the cat's environment is also driven by the impact of stressors on the cat's health. For example, the initial management for feline idiopathic cystitis now includes implementing environmental enrichment and methods to reduce stress.[41] The effect of cognitive enrichment on behavior, mucosal immunity and upper respiratory disease in a subgroup of shelter cats was recently studied.[42] Fifteen cats were labeled as "frustrated" based on behavioral characteristics in their cage, such as pacing, destructive behavior, persistent vocalization, bar biting, and escape trials.[42] Training sessions (10 minutes) using a clicker and food rewards to teach 8 cats to do a "high-five" were done 4 times daily over a 10-day period.[42] The other 7 cats were not trained.[42] The authors showed that cognitive enrichment in these cats compared with the untrained cats could elicit positive affect ("contentment"), stimulate intestinal immunoglobulin A secretion and reduce the incidence of upper respiratory disease.[42] Provision of cognitive enrichment for pet cats would probably require training sessions of at least 5 to 10 minutes daily. The cat would, thus, benefit from total attention from the owner, would be mentally stimulated, and rewarded with preferred food items. Offering choice to cats not only applies to individuals with behavior disorders, but to all cats, particularly the strictly indoor cats.

Once management strategies are in place, desensitization and counterconditioning can take place to change the pet's emotional state in response to a trigger stimulus (see Leslie Sinn's article, "Advances in Behavioral Psychopharmacology," in this issue).

TYPES OF TRAINING AND TOOLS

Traditional training methods have relied on positive punishment (a behavior or response is reduced by application of an aversive stimulus during or immediately within 1–3 seconds of the behavior) and negative reinforcement (a response or behavior is strengthened by stopping, removing, or avoiding a negative outcome or aversive stimulus).[43] In both cases, the animal is subjected to coercion and aversive events. In negative reinforcement, one must apply positive punishment first so that there will be an aversive stimulus to remove.[44] In contrast, negative punishment (removal of what the animal wants such as toys, treats, petting, or attention during the undesirable behavior) and positive reinforcement (food, toys, play, petting, or attention immediately after a desirable behavior) are neither coercive nor painful.

Dog Owner Surveys

A survey of 192 dog owners suggested that the use of punishment (verbal telling off, scruff, shake, or smack the dog) resulted in an increase of avoidance, fear, and aggression.[45] Inconsistency in training methods (use of positive punishment and positive reinforcement) was associated with the highest aggression scores.[45] A survey of 140 dog owners seeking appointments with a veterinary behaviorist to treat their dog's behavior problem showed that direct confrontational (ie, "alpha roll," "dominance down," hit or kick the dog, grab the jowls or scruff, knee the dog in the chest, remotely activated shock collar, etc) and indirect confrontational (yell "no," spray with water pistol or spray bottle, growl at dog, "stare down," etc) training methods were associated with aggressive behavior.[46] Behaviors such as hitting or kicking the dog, physically forcing the release of an item from the dog's mouth, alpha rolls, staring at or staring down the dog, "dominance down," or grabbing the dog by the jowls and shaking elicited an aggressive response in at least one-fourth of the dogs.[46] Owners are, thus, potentially at risk of aggression when using confrontational techniques to train their dogs. In contrast, using neutral (ie, avoidance, synthetic pheromones, exercise) or reward-based (ie, food rewards, clicker training, food-stuffed toys) methods was rarely associated with aggressive behaviors.[46] A survey of 1276 dog owners showed that higher frequencies of punishment were associated with higher aggression and excitability (all dogs) and fearfulness and anxiety (in small dogs).[47] Punishment consisted of scolding the dog verbally and jerking the leash (80% of the owners) and slapping the dog, grasping it around the muzzle, and shaking it by the scruff (30% of the owners).[47] A survey of 3897 dog owners showed that the use of positive punishment and negative reinforcement (citronella bark collar or remotely activated citronella collar, shouting, electric fence, electric collar, choke chain, prong collar, smacking, jerking back on lead, etc) was related to an increase in aggression between dogs in the household (3.8 times more likely) and aggression toward dogs outside the household (2.5 times more likely).[48] The use of positive punishment and negative reinforcement was related to an increase in aggression toward family members (2.9 times increased risk) and unfamiliar people outside of the house (2.2 times increased risk).[49] A survey of 326 dog owners suggested that reward-based training methods (play, food, praise, other unspecified methods) were associated with both higher levels of obedience and fewer behavior problems.[50] The reward frequency correlated positively with the summed obedience score.[50] Highest obedience scores were obtained by owners using reward-based methods only as opposed to a combination of punishment-based (smacking, tapping nose, shouting, tugging back on leash in heel training) and reward training or those using punishment only.[50] Another survey also reported more successful outcomes for owners using reward-based methods for training recall than those using electronic collars.[51]

These results, therefore, suggest that punishment-based training does not result in superior training performance. However, correlation does not necessarily mean causation. Therefore, as stated by several authors in various publications as cited, one can question whether the dog's aggression or behavior problem led to the use of aversive training methods or if the use of aversive training methods caused the aggression and other problems.

Observation of Dogs During Training

Rooney and Cowan[52] published that dogs trained with physical punishment were less likely to approach a stranger and played less with their owners. Physical punishment included use of choke chain or pinch collar, squirt water in the face, rub nose in feces, yank back, lift dog using collar, flick on the ear, and shake the dog.[52] Dogs that were mostly trained with reward-based methods (praise, food, play, clicker) scored higher in their ability to learn a novel task.[52] Deldalle and Gaunet[53] found that dogs trained with negative reinforcement showed more stress-related behaviors (mouth licking, yawning, shivering, scratching, sniffing, and whining) and lowered body postures, whereas dogs trained with positive reinforcement showed increased attentiveness to the owner. Military dogs that received more aversive stimuli (positive punishment or negative reinforcement) such as pulling on the leash, hanging the dog by the collar, verbal scolding, and hitting were more distracted and showed poorer performance than dogs with less aversive training methods.[54] These dogs showed a lowered posture after receiving the aversive stimulus (pulling on the leash or hanging the dogs by their collar).[54]

Electronic Collars

A study looked at behavioral and physiologic measures of 63 dogs in 3 groups (group A with trainers using e-collars, group B with the same trainers not using e-collars, and group C with trainers using reward-based training).[55] Group A dogs spent more time tense, yawned more frequently, and explored less than group C dogs.[55] There was no significant owner-reported difference in efficacy across groups.[55] Owners of group A dogs were less confident applying the training approach shown.[55] The study also showed evidence of a relationship between vocalizations and collar settings for group A, with yelping and all vocalizations increasing in parallel with average collar stimulus intensity setting across training days.[55] Finally, dogs in groups A and B required twice as many commands per training session than group C dogs.[55] This finding study suggested there were no consistent benefits using electronic collars during training and greater welfare concerns compared with positive reward-based training.[55] Dogs trained with shock collars in another study learned that the presence of the owner announced reception of shock, even outside the training context.[56] Direct reaction to shocks resulted in lowered body posture; high-pitched yelps, barks, and squeals; avoidance; redirected aggression; and tongue flicking.[56] These signs are compatible with fear and/or pain. In another study, poor timing for the application of high-level electrical pulses increased the risk of dogs experiencing severe and persistent signs of stress (physiologic measures).[57] Dogs can therefore be emotionally affected (fearful or stressed) by the use of shock collars both short and long term.[56,57] Another study also reported more vocal reactions elicited by the electronic collars than with pinch collars.[58]

Choke Collars

One case report describes injuries sustained by a German Shepherd disciplined and held above ground with a choke chain collar.[59] The neurologic examination revealed severe ischemic brain damage after strangulation.[59]

Regular Collar Versus Harness

Intraocular pressure was significantly increased from baseline values when a force was applied to the neck via a regular collar and leash but not when applied via a harness and leash.[60] "Slip collars," "choker collars," or other devices that varied in diameter when tension was applied were not used in this study.

Head Collar and Head Halter

Head collars or head halters have been described as tools for cases of aggressive behavior in the clinic. Various models exist and fit will vary from one dog to another, depending on anatomic characteristics of the dog's head and type of head collar used. Head collars generally give better control than other collar types over dogs that pull on leashes.[61]

Bark Collars

Citronella spray collars and electric shock collars were compared in 8 pet dogs for efficacy and user satisfaction.[62] Both collars were effective at reducing barking (88.9% for the citronella collar and 44% for the shock collar).[62] Seven owners out of 8 preferred the citronella collar (perceived as more humane) to the shock collar.[62] With the shock collar, some dogs made a painful cry and then continued barking.[62]

The most commonly reported problem with the citronella collar was an inappropriate discharge in response to noises other than the dog vocalizing.[62] Moffat and colleagues[63] found that citronella spray bark collars worn for 5 minutes were effective in reducing barking in 23 out of 30 dogs (76.7%) at the veterinary hospital. A scentless spray collar worn for 5 minutes was tested in 29 dogs and also resulted in reduction of barking in 17 of 29 dogs (58.6%).[63] Wells[64] reported that dogs generally habituated to the citronella spray bark collar when used for longer periods. A longer period of efficacy was noted if the collar was worn intermittently.[64] The efficacy of the citronella spray bark collars in 7 barking dogs was assessed.[65] Two dogs vocalizing when home alone responded differently to the collar.[65] One dog did not reduce vocalization (ie, the collar did not work) and the other dog no longer vocalized but instead hid under a veranda, trembling continuously during the trial of the collar.[65] These distress signs disappeared when the collar was removed.[65] Anecdotally, citronella collars are ineffective in dogs with separation-related vocalization, an anxiety disorder. The latter dog, likely suffering from separation anxiety, exhibited alternate signs of anxiety while wearing the citronella collar, because the spray collar does not address the underlying cause of the vocalization (ie, anxiety). The authors reported that the citronella collar was effective at reducing the vocalization in 3 of 7 dogs, but also stated that, for some dogs, the initial reduction in vocalization was not maintained with continued use.[65] Several owners reported that the collar was oversensitive to extraneous stimuli such as head shaking, vigorous movement, and panting.[65] The dogs were, therefore, sometimes sprayed in the absence of vocalization.[65]

Taking all these data into consideration, there is no scientific evidence to justify the use of electric shock collars over spray collars to reduce barking. Spray collars may be of help to decrease barking, because it is contingent with the unwanted behavior. However, like with any other behavioral complaints, it is important to go to the root of the problem and address the underlying motivation for barking and address it.

Basket Muzzle

Basket muzzles are the preferred muzzle style for behavior patients because, unlike muzzles that keep the mouth closed tight, they allow the dog to pant, eat, and drink. Dogs can, therefore, wear them for extended periods, within reason. Dogs can learn to wear a basket muzzle initially at home when they are calm. Several protocols are described using positive reinforcement and some are even available on YouTube.

MEDICATION

Psychotropic medication is prescribed to decrease reactivity and anxiety in addition to management and a behavioral modification plan. The veterinarian must have a complete history to make an appropriate drug choice, be able to objectively assess progress and have realistic expectations (prognosis). All of these aspects should be discussed with the pet owner before prescribing.

Behavioral History

The context, behavioral sequence, frequency, and severity (or duration) of the abnormal behavior are needed, as well as the occurrences of anxiety or stress-related behaviors. Take, for example, the dog that barks at unfamiliar dogs and unfamiliar people. Relevant questions should include the frequency in each context. The dog meets an unfamiliar dog but reacts 5 out of 10 times. This same dog meets an unfamiliar person during walks and reacts 10 times out of 10. Questions dealing specifically with reactivity should also be asked: Does the dog exhibit piloerection? Does the dog remain calm enough that he can "hear" the owner during the undesirable behavior? How long does it take the dog to recover after an event? Does the dog startle easily with benign sounds or movements? These data will allow the veterinarian to follow-up objectively on the efficacy of the medication with regard, in this example, to the reactivity and frequency of barking. Also, when discussing the problematic behavior with the owner, the veterinarian may realize that the context or triggers are easily avoidable. In such cases, drug therapy may not be necessary.[66]

Drug Choice

The next question is whether the animal is affected daily or situationally. Some medications, like anxiolytics, are fast acting, whereas most antidepressants may take weeks before full clinical effects are seen. Most of the time, owners are able to decrease exposure to triggers and the delayed clinical onset of the medication will not be problematic. However, in some situations, such as thunderstorm phobia and separation anxiety, rapid pharmacologic intervention may be required to ease the distress of the pet.

Ease of administration may influence the choice or formulation of the medication prescribed. Some drugs are given only once daily and others twice daily or more. Some drugs can be compounded in a liquid form or flavored chews. Bioavailability of transdermal fluoxetine in cats is lower than the value of oral administration in healthy individuals.[67,68] Dermal irritation at the site of application is possible after several days of transdermal fluoxetine treatment.[67,68]

With the exception of clomipramine (Clomicalm) for separation anxiety in dogs, selegiline (Anipryl) for cognitive dysfunction in dogs, and dexmedetomidine (Sileo) for noise aversion in dogs, use of psychotropic medication in pets is off-label. Fluoxetine (Reconcile) was approved for separation anxiety in dogs, but is no longer available. Therefore, when making a drug choice for cognitive dysfunction or separation anxiety in dogs, selegiline and clomipramine, respectively, should be the first options. It is the clinician's responsibility to inform the clients about off-label use of medication and what it implies for their pet.

Veterinary practitioners seeking for more information on appropriate drug choices for abnormal behaviors can refer to Leslie Sinn's article "Advances in Behavioral Psychopharmacology," in this issue, as well as various behavioral medicine textbooks and articles.[69–74]

Expectations

Setting realistic expectations with the owner is essential for success. With medication, reactivity should decrease and the animal should be able to hear owner instructions, recover faster after an event, not startle as easily, and so on. The veterinarian needs to also make sure that the owner understands the difference between control and cure of the behavior disorder.[66] For example, a fearfully aggressive dog may never be comfortable if touched suddenly by an unfamiliar person on the street. However, this dog may learn to walk by strangers without lunging at them. If the owner expected his or her dog to tolerate physical contact from strangers, he or she may be disappointed with the outcome. If the veterinarian validates the owner's expectations and ensures that they are realistic, disappointment will be avoided.

Owners should also be given an idea of the time frame necessary for changes. Most antidepressants require several weeks before clinical effects are observed. Adjusting the appropriate dosage also may require several weeks. Veterinary practitioners must be familiar with and able to explain clearly the side effects and undesirable interactions possible with other drugs the animal may be taking concurrently. Owners must be informed. Starting at the low end of the therapeutic range can help to mitigate any undesirable effects.[70]

SUMMARY

When presented with a behavioral complaint, veterinarians must identify all contributing medical or behavioral disorders. Veterinarians can give valuable information regarding management and training tools. Owners should be directed to trainers or staff who are familiar with positive, reward-based training techniques. Psychotropic medication is prescribed to animals with a behavioral disorder (abnormal behavior), showing signs of anxiety and/or increased reactivity. Veterinarians need to collect a thorough behavioral history, understand the rationale behind the use of a drug class, and discuss realistic expectations with pet owners.

REFERENCES

1. Sueda KLC, Malamed R. Canine aggression toward people: a guide for practitioners. Vet Clin North Am Small Anim Pract 2014;44:599–628.
2. Neilson JC. Feline house soiling: elimination and marking behaviors. Vet Clin North Am Small Anim Pract 2003;33:287–301.
3. Landsberg G, Hunthausen W, Ackerman L. Stereotypic and compulsive disorders. In: Landsberg G, Hunthausen W, Ackerman L, editors. Behavior problems of the dog & cat. 3rd edition. Edinburgh (UK): Saunders Elsevier; 2013. p. 163–79.
4. Bécuwe-Bonnet V, Bélanger MC, Frank D, et al. Gastrointestinal disorders in dogs with excessive licking of surfaces. J Vet Behav Clin Appl Res 2012;7(4):194–204.
5. Frank D, Bélanger MC, Bécuwe-Bonnet V, et al. Prospective medical evaluation of 7 dogs presented with fly biting. Can Vet J 2012;53:1279–84.
6. Poirier-Guay M-P, Bélanger M-C, Frank D. Star gazing in a dog: atypical manifestation of upper gastrointestinal disease. Can Vet J 2014;55:1079–82.
7. Dinan TG, Cryan JF. Regulation of the stress response by the gut microbiota: implications for psychoneuroendocrinology. Psychoneuroendocrinology 2012;37: 1369–78.
8. Sherwin E, Rea K, Dinan TG, et al. A gut (microbiome) feeling about the brain. Curr Opin Gastroenterol 2016;32:96–102.
9. Sampson TR, Mazmanian SK. Control of brain development, function, and behavior by the microbiome. Cell Host Microbe 2015;17:565–76.
10. Bellono NW, Bayrer JR, Leitch DB, et al. Enterochromaffin cells are gut chemosensors that couple to sensory neural pathways. Cell 2017;170:185–98, e116.
11. Clarke G, Stilling RM, Kennedy PJ, et al. Minireview: gut microbiota: the neglected endocrine organ. Mol Endocrinol 2014;28:1221–38.
12. Virga V. Behavioral dermatology. Vet Clin North Am 2003;33:231–51.
13. Horwitz DF, Neilson JC. Blackwell's five-minute veterinary consult clinical companion: canine and feline behavior. Chapter 39 (Psychogenic alopecia/overgrooming: feline). Ames (IA): Blackwell Publishing; 2007. p. 425–31.
14. Waisglass SE, Landsberg GM, Yager JA, et al. Underlying medical conditions in cats with presumptive psychogenic alopecia. J Am Vet Med Assoc 2006;228: 1705–9.
15. Garg A, Chren M-M, Sands LP, et al. Psychological stress perturbs epidermal permeability barrier homeostasis: implications for the pathogenesis of stress-associated skin disorders. Arch Dermatol 2001;137:53–9.
16. Denda M, Tsuchiya T, Elias PM, et al. Stress alters cutaneous permeability barrier homeostasis. Am J Physiol Regul Integr Comp Physiol 2000;278:R367–72.

17. Landsberg G, Hunthausen W, Ackerman L. Behavior problems of the dog & cat. 3rd edition. Edinburgh (UK): Saunders Elsevier; 2013. p. 75–94.

18. Nagata M, Shibata K. Importance of psychogenic factors in canine recurrent pyoderma. Vet Dermatol 2004;15:42.

19. Dreschel NA. The effects of fear and anxiety on health and lifespan in pet dogs. Appl Anim Behav Sci 2010;125:157–62.

20. Mazur JE. History, background, and basic concepts. In: Mazur JE, editor. Learning and behavior. 7th edition. New York: Psychology Press Taylor & Francis Group; 2013. p. 1–25.

21. Horwitz DF, Pike AL. Common sense behavior modification: a guide for practitioners. Vet Clin North Am Small Anim Pract 2014;44:401–26.

22. Voith VL, Borchelt PL. Diagnosis and treatment of dominance aggression in dogs. Vet Clin North Am Small Anim Pract 1982;12:655–63.

23. Overall KL. Protocol for deference. In: Overall KL, editor. Manual of clinical behavioral medicine for dogs and cats. St Louis (MO): Elsevier Mosby; 2013. p. 574–9.

24. Yin S. Dominance versus leadership in dog training. Compend Contin Educ Vet 2007;29:414.

25. Voith VL, Ingram E, Mitsouras K, et al. Comparison of adoption agency breed identification and DNA breed identification of dogs. J Appl Anim Welf Sci 2009; 12:253–62.

26. Voith VL, Trevejo R, Dowling-Guyer S, et al. Comparison of visual and DNA breed identification of dogs and inter-observer reliability. Am J Socio Res 2013;3:17–29.

27. Reisner IR, Nance ML, Zeller JS, et al. Behavioural characteristics associated with dog bites to children presenting to an urban trauma centre. Inj Prev 2011;17(5):348–53.

28. Reisner IR, Shofer FS, Nance ML. Behavioral assessment of child-directed canine aggression. Inj Prev 2007;13:348–51.

29. Reisner IR, Shofer FS. Effects of gender and parental status on knowledge and attitudes of dog owners regarding dog aggression toward children. J Am Vet Med Assoc 2008;233:1412–9.

30. Kahn A, Bauche P, Lamoureux J, et al. Child victims of dog bites treated in emergency departments: a prospective survey. Eur J Pediatr 2003;162:254–8.

31. Chapman S, Cornwall J, Righetti J, et al. Preventing dog bites in children: randomised controlled trial of an educational intervention. BMJ 2000;320:1512–3.

32. Hart B, Barrett R. Effects of castration on fighting, roaming, and urine spraying in adult male cats. J Am Vet Med Assoc 1973;163:290–2.

33. Hart B, Cooper L. Factors relating to urine spraying and fighting in prepubertally gonadectomized cats. J Am Vet Med Assoc 1984;184:1255–8.

34. Hopkins S, Schubert T, Hart B. Castration of adult male dogs: effects on roaming, aggression, urine marking, and mounting. J Am Vet Med Assoc 1976;168:1108–10.

35. Neilson JC, Eckstein RA, Hart B. Effects of castration on problem behaviors in male dogs with reference to age and duration of behavior. J Am Vet Med Assoc 1997;211:180–2.

36. Horwitz DF, Neilson JC. Blackwell's five-minute veterinary consult clinical companion canine and feline behavior. Ames (IA): Blackwell Publishing; 2007. p. 10–7.

37. Stella JL, Croney CC. Environmental aspects of domestic cat care and management: implications for cat welfare. ScientificWorldJournal 2016;2016:6296315.

38. Ellis SL. Environmental enrichment: practical strategies for improving feline welfare. J Feline Med Surg 2009;11:901–12.

39. Heath S, Wilson C. Canine and feline enrichment in the home and kennel. Vet Clin North Am Small Anim Pract 2014;44:427–49.

40. Ellis J, Stryhn H, Spears J, et al. Environmental enrichment choices of shelter cats. Behav Processes 2017;141(Pt 3):291–6.

41. Forrester SD, Towell TL. Feline idiopathic cystitis. Vet Clin North Am Small Anim Pract 2015;45:783–806.

42. Gourkow N, Phillips CJ. Effect of cognitive enrichment on behavior, mucosal immunity and upper respiratory disease of shelter cats rated as frustrated on arrival. Prev Vet Med 2016;131:103–10.

43. Landsberg G, Hunthausen W, Ackerman L. Handbook of behavior problems of the dog and the cat. 2nd edition. Edinburgh (UK): Saunders Elsevier; 2003. p. 91–116.

44. Ziv G. The effects of using aversive training methods in dogs – a review. J Vet Behav Clin Appl Res 2017;19:50–60.

45. Blackwell EJ, Twells C, Seawright A, et al. The relationship between training methods and the occurrence of behavior problems, as reported by owners, in a population of domestic dogs. J Vet Behav Clin Appl Res 2008;3:207–17.

46. Herron ME, Shofer FS, Reisner IR. Survey of the use and outcome of confrontational and non-confrontational training methods in client-owned dogs showing undesired behaviors. Appl Anim Behav Sci 2009;117:47–54.

47. Arhant C, Bubna-Littitz H, Bartels A, et al. Behaviour of smaller and larger dogs: effects of training methods, inconsistency of owner behaviour and level of engagement in activities with the dog. Appl Anim Behav Sci 2010;123:131–42.

48. Casey R, Loftus B, Bolster C, et al. Inter-dog aggression in a UK owner survey: prevalence, co-occurrence in different contexts and risk factors. Vet Rec 2013; 172:127.

49. Casey RA, Loftus B, Bolster C, et al. Human directed aggression in domestic dogs (Canis familiaris): occurrence in different contexts and risk factors. Appl Anim Behav Sci 2014;152:52–63.

50. Hiby E, Rooney N, Bradshaw J. Dog training methods: their use, effectiveness and interaction with behaviour and welfare. Anim Welf 2004;13:63–70.

51. Blackwell EJ, Bolster C, Richards G, et al. The use of electronic collars for training domestic dogs: estimated prevalence, reasons and risk factors for use, and owner perceived success as compared to other training methods. BMC Vet Res 2012;8:93.

52. Rooney NJ, Cowan S. Training methods and owner–dog interactions: links with dog behaviour and learning ability. Appl Anim Behav Sci 2011;132:169–77.

53. Deldalle S, Gaunet F. Effects of 2 training methods on stress-related behaviors of the dog (Canis familiaris) and on the dog–owner relationship. J Vet Behav Clin Appl Res 2014;9:58–65.

54. Haverbeke A, Laporte B, Depiereux E, et al. Training methods of military dog handlers and their effects on the team's performances. Appl Anim Behav Sci 2008; 113:110–22.

55. Cooper JJ, Cracknell N, Hardiman J, et al. The welfare consequences and efficacy of training pet dogs with remote electronic training collars in comparison to reward based training. PLoS One 2014;9:e102722.

56. Schilder MB, van der Borg JA. Training dogs with help of the shock collar: short and long term behavioural effects. Appl Anim Behav Sci 2004;85:319–34.

57. Schalke E, Stichnoth J, Ott S, et al. Clinical signs caused by the use of electric training collars on dogs in everyday life situations. Appl Anim Behav Sci 2007; 105:369–80.

58. Salgirli Y, Schalke E, Boehm I, et al. Comparison of learning effects and stress between 3 different training methods (electronic training collar, pinch collar and quitting signal) in Belgian Malinois Police Dogs. Revue Méd Vét 2012;163:530–5.

59. Grohmann K, Dickomeit MJ, Schmidt MJ, et al. Severe brain damage after punitive training technique with a choke chain collar in a German shepherd dog. J Vet Behav Clin Appl Res 2013;8:180–4.
60. Pauli AM, Bentley E, Diehl KA, et al. Effects of the application of neck pressure by a collar or harness on intraocular pressure in dogs. J Am Anim Hosp Assoc 2006; 42:207–11.
61. Moffat K. Addressing canine and feline aggression in the veterinary clinic. Vet Clin North Am Small Anim Pract 2008;38:983–1003.
62. Juarbe-Diaz S, Houpt K, Hikasa Y, et al. Comparison of two antibarking collars for treatment of nuisance barking. J Am Anim Hosp Assoc 1996;32:231–5.
63. Moffat KS, Landsberg GM, Beaudet R. Effectiveness and comparison of citronella and scentless spray bark collars for the control of barking in a veterinary hospital setting. J Am Anim Hosp Assoc 2003;39:343–8.
64. Wells DL. The effectiveness of a citronella spray collar in reducing certain forms of barking in dogs. Appl Anim Behav Sci 2001;73:299–309.
65. Sargisson RJ, Butler R, Elliffe D. An evaluation of the Aboistop citronella-spray collar as a treatment for barking of domestic dogs. ISRN Vet Sci 2012;2011: 759379.
66. Seibert LM, Landsberg GM. Diagnosis and management of patients presenting with behavior problems. Vet Clin North Am Small Anim Pract 2008;38:937–50.
67. Ciribassi J, Luescher A, Pasloske KS, et al. Comparative bioavailability of fluoxetine after transdermal and oral administration to healthy cats. Am J Vet Res 2003;64:994–8.
68. Eichstadt L, Corriveau L, Moore G, et al. Absorption of transdermal fluoxetine compounded in a lipoderm base compared to oral fluoxetine in client-owned cats. Int J Pharm Compd 2017;21:242.
69. Landsberg G, Hunthausen W, Ackerman L. Behavior problems of the dog & cat. 3rd edition. Edinburgh (UK): Saunders Elsevier; 2013.
70. Simpson BS, Papich MG. Pharmacologic management in veterinary behavioral medicine. Vet Clin North Am Small Anim Pract 2003;33:365–404.
71. Horwitz DF, Neilson JC. Blackwell's five-minute veterinary consult clinical companion: canine and feline behavior. Ames (IA): Blackwell Publishing; 2007.
72. Crowell-Davis SL, Murray T. Veterinary psychopharmacology. Ames (IA): John Wiley & Sons; 2008.
73. Horwitz D, Mills D. BSAVA manual of canine and feline behavioural medicine. Quedgeley, Gloucester (UK): BSAVA; 2009.
74. Overall KL. Manual of clinical behavioral medicine for dogs and cats. St Louis (MO): Mosby Elsevier; 2013.

Separation, Confinement, or Noises: What Is Scaring That Dog?

Kelly C. Ballantyne, DVM*

KEYWORDS

- Canine • Separation anxiety • Noise aversion • Noise phobia
- Behavior modification

KEY POINTS

- Separation anxiety and noise aversions are significant welfare issues that affect many companion dogs.
- Video is key in the diagnosis of separation anxiety and in differentiating it from confinement distress and noise aversions.
- Treatment of these conditions using a combination of psychopharmaceuticals and behavior modification is recommended to improve welfare as quickly as possible.

INTRODUCTION

Separation anxiety and noise aversions are 2 of the most common behavioral disorders of dogs with approximately 17% to 29% reported to have separation anxiety[1–3] and 23% to 49% reported to have noise aversion.[1,4–6] These conditions can be comorbid with each other and with other fear-related behavioral disorders.[1,4,7–10] Separation anxiety and noise aversions present significant welfare issues for affected dogs; they cause emotional distress, can interfere with normal functioning, may result in self-trauma, and increase the dog's risk of relinquishment or euthanasia. These conditions can also negatively impact the quality of life of the pet owner or owners.[11] Identification and prompt treatment are needed to reduce suffering.

Terminology

The fear emotion is highly conserved across species and evolved to detect threats and initiate the behavioral and physiologic response needed to survive them. Animals learn which stimuli to fear through an unconscious process called fear conditioning. Fear conditioning is highly resistant to forgetting because it is critical to remember which environmental stimuli are safe and which are unsafe; however, fear conditioning can

Disclosure Statement: The author has nothing to disclose.
Veterinary Clinical Medicine, University of Illinois College of Veterinary Medicine, Urbana, IL, USA
* 2242 West Harrison Street Suite 101, Chicago, IL 60612.
E-mail address: kcmorgan@illinois.edu

lead to learning that innocuous or neutral stimuli are unsafe, resulting in chronic emotional distress.[12] Anxieties, fears, and phobias refer to emotional, behavioral, and physiologic responses to threatening stimuli. Although these terms are sometimes used interchangeably, they refer to different emotional states and may have different neurobiological mechanisms.[13]

- Anxiety is anticipation of a danger or threat. The stimulus for the response is not always identifiable or present.
- Fear is an emotional, behavioral, and physiologic response to a stimulus that the animal perceives is threatening.
- Phobia is a persistent and maladaptive fear that is out of proportion to the situation or stimulus.[14]

Signs of Fear in Dogs

Signs of fear in dogs can be active or passive and include avoidance or hiding, flattened ears, lowered body posture, low tail position, pacing or excessive activity, visual scanning/hypervigilance, seeking out contact with humans and other animals, and aggression. Physiologic signs of fear in dogs include panting, salivation, urination and defecation, tense muscles, dilated pupils, and anorexia.[15,16] Dogs that have separation-related distress, confinement distress, or noise aversions will show similar clinical signs, and these conditions can be confused with each other.[13,17] Identifying the stimuli or conditions that elicit these signs is important in differentiating separation anxiety, confinement distress, and noise aversions from each other and for identifying comorbidity[10,14] **(Table 1)**.

Separation Anxiety

Separation-related behaviors are described with terms including separation anxiety, separation-related disorder, and separation-related distress. Although this is the most well studied behavioral disorder in dogs, there is no consensus on diagnostic terminology.[13] The term separation anxiety is used throughout this article to describe dogs that show signs of distress when separated from the person or persons to whom they are most attached or when left alone without a human companion. The diagnostic criteria for separation anxiety are that signs occur only when the dog is alone or cannot access its owner.[2,20] Separation anxiety signs may be shown in the absence or perceived absence of the owner or owners—some dogs will become distressed if the owner is in an area of the home that the dog cannot access.[2,14] The most common owner complaints of dogs with separation anxiety are house soiling, destruction, and excessive vocalization[3,8,17,21–23]; dogs that experience distress but whose signs do not leave evidence (ie, pacing, panting, whining) may go undiagnosed. Having another dog in the house does not prevent separation anxiety,[10] and video analysis shows that affected dogs that live with other dogs behave similarly to affected dogs that live alone.[21] Dogs may show signs of distress within 10 to 30 minutes of the owner's departure,[21,24] and signs of separation anxiety typically occur every time the dog is home alone regardless of the duration of the owner's absence.[14,20] Some owners may report signs occur only occasionally or when the dog is left alone outside of its normal routine,[24] but these inconsistent reactions to being left alone may reflect an intensification of the dog's distress following routine changes[25] rather than inconsistent distress, or may indicate the presence of a comorbid condition such as noise aversion.[19] For example, some dogs may pace, pant, and whine or remain vigilant whenever home alone but may bark repeatedly and destroy items when alone off-routine or during storms. Without

Table 1
Signs and triggers

Signs[15,16,18]			Triggers		
Active	Passive	Physiologic	Separation-Related Distress	Confinement Distress	Noise Aversion
• Pacing, running, or circling • Digging or clawing • Chewing or destruction • Climbing • Jumping • Barking • Aggression	• Hiding • Crouching, cowering, tucked tail • Ears turned back • Alert, vigilant • Lip licking • Foreleg lift • Whining	• Salivation • Tense muscles • Urination or defecation • Panting • Trembling • Dilated pupils • Anorexia	• Owner preparing to leave • Owner's physical or virtual absence • Owner's return home	• Confinement regardless of owner's presence or absence	• Loud noises (ie, fireworks, thunder, gunshots, construction equipment) • Stimuli associated with loud noises (ie, flashing lights, rain, dark skies)
Owners may note a combination of active, passive, and physiologic signs			When these conditions are comorbid, signs of distress intensify when events combine (ie, separation + confinement; separation + loud noise event)[7,19]		

video, the owner only finds evidence of the more intense responses. Video analysis of dogs with separation anxiety shows that affected dogs spend most of their time oriented to the environment—sitting or lying down with head up and looking around[21]—whereas unaffected dogs spend most of their time resting or sleeping.[26] When destructive behavior occurs, it is often targeted at exit points, and severely affected dogs can cause significant property damage in their efforts to restore contact with the owner or escape the home (**Fig. 1**). Many dogs with separation anxiety show signs of distress as the owner prepares to leave the house[8,10,17,24] and show excessive enthusiasm or increased activity upon the owner's return.[8,17,27] Unaffected dogs may also appear excited when the owner returns home and may greet more intensely following longer separations,[28] but dogs with separation anxiety are more likely to show excessive greeting behaviors or increased activity regardless of the duration of the owner's absence.[8,27] Subsets of dogs with separation anxiety may appear excessively "needy," remaining within sight of their owner most of the day,[8] but this type of behavior is not seen in all dogs with separation anxiety and is not a necessary diagnostic criteria.[24,29,30] There is no consistent agreement in risk factors such as age, breed, and owner-related factors among studies that looked for them.[13]

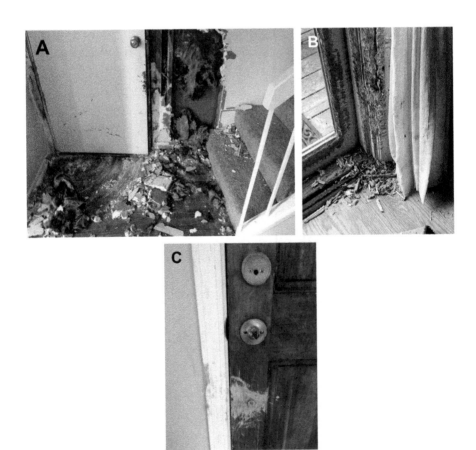

Fig. 1. (*A–C*) The metal doorknob and lock on this door were chewed off by a dog with separation anxiety.

Video analysis of dogs with separation anxiety
A study that used video to analyze separation anxiety found that dogs spent most of their time oriented to the environment or vigilant, but barking and vigilance decreased with time, whereas panting tended to increase with time. This study also identified 3 different types of responses to being home alone[21]:

- Discomfort response: lip licking, yawning, paw raised
- Fearful response: increased motor activity and escape or decreased motor behavior/behavioral inhibition
- Anxious response: increased attention to environment, vocalization, decreased exploration

These different response types may represent different underlying emotional states in the affected dogs and may explain discrepancies in recommendations on how to treat separation anxiety as well as treatment failures.[21]

Confinement Distress

Confinement distress is used to describe dogs that show anxiety, fear, or panic when confined in a crate, kennel, or small room. Although little work has been done to investigate confinement distress in dogs, one study of dogs with separation anxiety showed that confined dogs yawned and licked their lips more than unconfined dogs,[21] possibly indicating a higher intensity of anxiety in confined dogs. Other studies show no direct correlation between confinement and separation anxiety,[10,26,31] which suggests that confinement distress is a separate disorder. Confinement distress is observed in dogs when they are confined regardless of the owner's presence,[14,32] but signs may be more intense when the dog is confined during distressing events (ie, confined while home alone or during fireworks). Dogs that panic during confinement show intense escape-behaviors, bending metal crate bars with their teeth, paws, or body or chewing through plastic crates. Some owners may report coming home to find the dog out of its crate with the crate door still closed. Dogs with only confinement distress may tolerate separation from their owners if not confined, but dogs with both confinement distress and separation anxiety and/or noise aversion may house soil or destroy items when home alone or during noise events. Owners may increase their efforts to confine the dog to prevent property damage, purchasing "escape-proof" crates or securing the crates with cords or locks. Forcing confinement heightens the dog's panic and escalates intensity of escape-behaviors, resulting in self-trauma and in severe cases death (**Fig. 2**). Dogs with either separation anxiety or confinement distress may show signs when confined at the groomer, boarding and daycare facilities, and veterinary hospitals/clinics. Confinement distress is ruled out if the dog voluntarily seeks out its confinement area for a resting spot.[32]

Noise Aversions

Noise aversion is a general term to describe anxious, fearful, or phobic responses to noises. This term is used in lieu of noise phobia throughout this article because many dogs do not meet the noise phobia diagnostic criteria: a profound, nongraded, and extreme response to noise.[2,7,14,33] Common signs of noise aversions in dogs include trembling, freezing, panting, social withdrawal, pacing, salivation, urination, defecation, destruction, hiding, crouching, and escape behaviors.[2,5,6,14,33] Destruction and escape behaviors may cause self-injury.[6] The most frequent trigger for noise aversions in dogs is fireworks, but other common triggers include thunder, gunfire, and noises from motor vehicles.[2,4,5] Noise aversions may be stimulus specific,[33] only occurring in response to one type of noise (ie, fireworks); can generalize to noises with similar characteristics (ie, fireworks and gunfire)[4,5]; can generalize to conditions that frequently cooccur with the

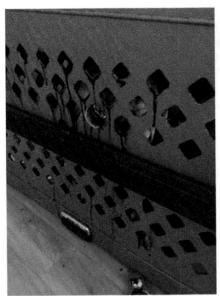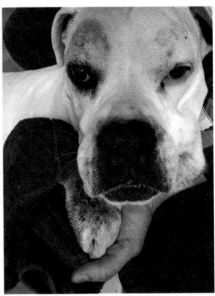

Fig. 2. This dog's mandible was trapped in the side of this metal crate and firefighters had to assist in cutting her free. Note the blood and injured forepaw.

loud noise (ie, dark skies, flashing lights, rain, wind), or the location in which the loud noise was experienced. Dogs with noise aversions may be fearful in novel situations and may take a longer time to calm down following a stressor compared with unaffected dogs.[4] Owners of dogs with noise aversions will observe signs of distress when they are with the dog during noise events, but signs may be more intense when the dog is alone during loud noise events—mimicking separation anxiety.[19] Possible factors contributing to the development of noise aversions include genetics, trauma associated with a noise, sensitization from the cumulative effect of repeated exposures, and social transmission.[34] Noise aversions present at any age but the risk or severity of signs may increase with age.[4–6] This condition can affect any breed, but sensitive breeds include shepherds, collies, and other herding dogs.[20] There may be breed-associated behavioral differences in the noise response—in a study that investigated behavioral responses to noises in German shepherds, Australian shepherds, and border collies, German shepherds were more likely to pace, whereas Australian shepherds and border collies were more likely to pant and hide.[33]

Comorbidity

Separation anxiety, confinement distress, or noise aversion may cooccur with each other or with other behavioral disorders, such as fear-related aggression or compulsive disorders. Several studies have reported a positive association between separation anxiety and noise aversions[4,7–9] as well as with other fear-related behaviors.[1,4] When presented with one of these conditions, it is important for clinicians to question dog owners about the dog's response to a range of situations to determine the presence of other behavioral disorders that may require treatment.

THE BEHAVIORAL HISTORY

Fear and anxiety disorders, like other illnesses, respond best to treatment when identified early, but many dogs that suffer from separation anxiety and noise aversions are untreated. One study reported that only 13% of owners whose dogs demonstrated separation-related behaviors sought professional advice.[3] As few as 16% to 29% of pet owners whose pets experience noise aversions may seek assistance.[5,6] Unfortunately, many dog owners may not know who to reach out to when their dog engages in problematic behaviors,[11] may not recognize all signs of fear and anxiety,[5,35] or may only reach out once the problem has escalated to the point of crisis. Open-ended questions, such as "what concerns do you have about your dog's behavior," can start a dialogue with the pet owner at every veterinary visit while gathering general health history. If behavioral concerns are noted, focused questions can help the veterinarian establish a diagnosis. The dog owner should be asked to give an objective description of the behavior—what the behavior looks like—or gather video to determine the characteristics of the problem and establish a baseline to measure treatment against. Questions about specific triggers for the dog's distress will help to determine the diagnosis as well as the most effective treatment plan. Goals of the behavioral history are to identify the following:

- An objective description of the behavior or behaviors
- Events or conditions that elicit the behavior or behaviors
- Intensity, duration, and frequency of the behavior or behaviors
- How the behavior resolves and how long it takes the dog to recover
- Owner responses to the behavior or behaviors

Table 2 lists specific examples.

DIFFERENTIAL DIAGNOSES

Medical differential diagnoses for fear and anxiety in dogs include neurologic disorders, conditions that cause chronic pain or discomfort, metabolic disorders, and sensory changes.[36] If house soiling is a presenting complaint, any condition or medication that results in increased frequency or urgency to eliminate, and any condition that causes pain on elimination, should be considered.[36] Detailed reviews of medical differentials for fear and anxiety are available.[16,37]

Separation anxiety, confinement distress, and noise aversions are differential diagnoses for each other. Noise aversions are typically straightforward to identify if the owner

Table 2
History questions

Separation-Related and Confinement Distress	Noise Aversion
• What behaviors are observed before the owner's departure?	• What does the dog do (what does the behavior look like)?
• What does the dog do when home alone? Video is essential to accurately answer this question.	• What noises does the dog respond to? • What noise-associated stimuli does the dog respond to?
• What does the dog do when the owner returns home?	• How long does it take the dog to return to baseline behavior/recover?
• What does the dog do when the owner is home/what percentage of the time is the dog within sight of the owner?	• Is the behavior same, better, or worse when the owner is present or absent?
• Where is the dog kept when home alone?	• How many noise events occur per week?
• If confinement is used, is the behavior same, better, or worse when confined vs unconfined?	• If confinement is used, is the behavior same, better, or worse when confined vs unconfined?

witnesses the dog's response to the noise. Behavioral differential diagnoses for separation anxiety include territorial behavior, play/unruly behavior, and cognitive dysfunction syndrome if the dog is 8 years of age or older. If house soiling is a presenting complaint, incomplete house training and urine marking should also be considered.[14]

Decisive Diagnostic Factors

- Separation-related distress: Signs of distress occur only when the dog is alone or in the perceived absence of the owner.[2,20]
- Confinement distress: Signs of distress occur when the dog is confined regardless of the owner's presence.[14,32]
- Noise aversions: Signs of distress occur in response a loud noise or noises.[14]

If these factors are unclear or mixed, video of the pet home alone will confirm the diagnosis or diagnoses.

PHYSICAL EXAMINATION AND DIAGNOSTICS

If signs of fear, anxiety, or distress are identified, a physical examination, complete blood count, chemistry profile, T4, and urinalysis should be performed to investigate for medical issues that may be causing or contributing to the problem. Dogs with separation anxiety, confinement distress, and noise aversions may present with injuries from escape attempts or destructive behavior, such as fractured crowns, broken nails on forepaws, and cuts and abrasions around muzzle, nose, or paws.

TREATMENT GOALS

Treatment of separation anxiety, confinement distress, and noise aversions is focused on reducing the intensity of dog's distress and improving its ability to function in its home environment.[14] Depending on the condition's severity or complexity, total resolution may not be possible and management may be a more realistic goal.[14,38]

PHARMACOLOGIC STRATEGIES

Separation anxiety and noise aversions often require pharmacologic treatment in addition to behavioral management strategies.[14] The goal of pharmacologic treatment is to reduce fear and anxiety as quickly as possible to improve the dog's welfare.[22,23] Although medications can help to relieve suffering and improve both the pet and the owner's welfare, there are several important issues to consider before prescribing a medication. In addition to evaluating the patient for physical conditions that may be causing or contributing to the behavioral problem—or may contraindicate certain medications—the animal's physical and social environment needs to be addressed with behavioral management strategies. Without addressing these issues, the patient's response to medication may be inadequate.[19,20,39] It is also important to discuss realistic expectations with the client when prescribing psychopharmaceuticals. Psychopharmaceuticals can reduce fear and arousal—resulting in a decrease in the severity, frequency, or intensity of the problem as well as improvement in recovery times—but complete elimination of fear or anxiety is unlikely.

Pharmaceutical Treatment of Separation Anxiety

Antidepressants

Fluoxetine (a selective serotonin reuptake inhibitor) and clomipramine (a tricyclic antidepressant) are effective for the treatment of separation anxiety with comparable results in placebo-controlled clinical trials.[22,23] The full therapeutic effects are achieved in 4 to 6 weeks, with some patients demonstrating signs of improvement as early as 1 week into treatment.[9,22] In one study that analyzed clomipramine treatment effect using video, dogs showed an increase in passive behavior (ie, resting) as early as week 1, with further increased passive behavior and reduction in barking in subsequent weeks and following an increase in clomipramine dose.[9] Fluoxetine also improved owner-rated separation anxiety severity scores when administered without a formal behavior modification plan.[40] Some investigators question whether these medications have an affect beyond their potential sedative side effects.[41] To investigate this issue in dogs treated for separation anxiety, a spatial cognitive bias test was used to determine if treatment with fluoxetine and behavior modification resulted in an improvement of the dog's emotional state or general motor inhibition.[42] Cognitive bias tests are used to investigate animals' affective (ie, emotional) states based on findings that an individual's background affective state biases its decision-making; individuals in negative states make more negative judgments about ambiguous stimuli than individuals in positive states.[43,44] In spatial cognitive bias tests, dogs are trained to discriminate between bowls placed in 2 different locations, one with food (positive location: P), and one without food (negative location: N). Once dogs learn to discriminate the 2 locations, placing bowls in ambiguous locations between the P and N locations tests their bias. An "optimistic" bias is rated in moving faster to the ambiguous locations, and a "pessimistic" bias is rated by moving slower to the ambiguous locations.[45] Dogs with separation anxiety showed a pessimistic bias compared with unaffected control dogs before treatment, but these differences disappeared by weeks 2 and 6—their cognitive bias normalized. Improvement in cognitive bias was also correlated with improvement in clinical measures of separation anxiety. This suggests that fluoxetine's treatment effect is related to an underlying improvement in affective state—its antidepressant effect—rather than behavioral inhibition.[42]

Rapidly acting anxiolytics
Rapidly acting anxiolytics may be used in severely affected pets when immediate control of separation anxiety is needed,[14] such as cases where the owner cannot avoid leaving the dog alone.

- Trazodone and clonidine may be administered 1 to 2 hours before owner's departures as needed.[46,47] Doses may be repeated with a minimum of 6 hours between doses of clonidine[47] and 8 hours between doses of trazodone.[48]
- Benzodiazepines, such as alprazolam and diazepam, may be administered situationally 1 hour before owner departure.[14] The frequency of redosing depends on the specific benzodiazepine prescribed.[49]

Combination therapy for separation anxiety
Combination therapy involves using medications with different pharmacologic mechanisms, dosing intervals, and onsets of effect. Combination therapy is used when[49]

- A rapid response to treatment is needed
- The patient does not respond sufficiently to one medication
- Side effects are noted as the dosage is increased
- Particularly panic-inducing situations are predicted

One strategy used early in separation anxiety treatment is using medications with complementary effects—administering a rapidly acting anxiolytic as needed before owner departures while administering the slower-onset antidepressant daily regardless of owner departures.[14] This strategy may reduce the dog's distress quickly before the antidepressant and behavior modification can take effect. In severely affected dogs, combination therapy may provide the most effective control of the dog's distress throughout treatment.[46,47] Although combination therapy is sometimes necessary in the treatment of separation anxiety and may help to prevent erosion of the human-animal bond, relinquishment or euthanasia combinations should be used cautiously. Clinicians should consider potential drug interactions as well as health risks before using combination therapy. During treatment, patients should be monitored closely for desired effects and side effects.[49,50] If the patient is not responding to treatment as expected, its health status should be reassessed along with the management and behavior modification plan.

Pharmaceutical Treatment of Noise Aversions

The type of medication selected for treatment of noise aversions will depend on the frequency of noise events in the dog's environment as well as the intensity of the dog's response to the noise.[20]

- Dogs that experience infrequent noise events and whose signs are consistent with fear or anxiety may respond well to treatment with rapidly acting anxiolytics administered before predicted events.[51]
- Dogs that experience frequent noise events, dogs that exhibit signs of panic or phobia, or dogs with comorbidities such as separation anxiety or generalized anxiety benefit from treatment with an antidepressant, such as fluoxetine or clomipramine, in combination with rapidly acting anxiolytics.[14,20,34,38]
- For best effect when treating storm aversions, owners should be coached to monitor the weather and administer event medications when there is ≥50% chance of storms. It is better for the dog to receive the medication and not need it than need the medication and not get it and experience further sensitization to storms.[34]

Rapidly acting anxiolytics

As noted above, several as-needed medications are available to treat anxieties and fears. Sileo (dexmedetomidine oromucosal gel) is US Food and Drug Administration approved for the treatment of noise aversions in dogs. In a randomized, double-blind, placebo-controlled trial, Sileo demonstrated an excellent to good effect in 75% of treated dogs compared with an excellent to good effect in 33% of placebo dogs.[51]

- Sileo is administered situationally 15 to 60 minutes before a predicted noise event, at the first sign of fear, or when the owner detects a typical noise stimulus (eg, fireworks).
  - The dose may be repeated up to 5 times in 24 hours, with a minimum of 2 hours between doses.
- Benzodiazepines may be administered situationally 30 to 60 minutes before a predicted noise event.[14] The frequency of redosing depends on the specific benzodiazepine prescribed.[49]
  - Alprazolam (Xanax) is a good choice for noise aversions because of its rapid onset of effect (30 minutes), and anxiolysis is achieved at doses below those that result in sedation and ataxia.[38,49]
- Trazodone and clonidine may be administered situationally 1 to 2 hours before a predicted noise event.[46,47] Clonidine may be repeated with a minimum of 6 hours between doses,[47] and trazodone may be repeated with a minimum of 8 hours between doses.[48]

NONPHARMACEUTICAL TREATMENTS: BEHAVIORAL MANAGEMENT

Behavioral management strategies focus on avoidance of triggers, environmental modification to improve the dog's comfort, modification of dog-owner interactions, and behavior modification exercises to improve the dog's response to feared stimuli. **Table 3** provides examples on how to use these techniques for separation anxiety and noise aversion.

Compliance with Behavioral Management Strategies

Client compliance with treatment recommendations is a significant issue in veterinary behavior medicine.[24,52,53] Compliance may decline with the number of tasks assigned[53] or for methods that require a significant owner lifestyle change.[24,53] Although several behavior modification strategies are proposed for treatment of separation anxiety and noise phobia, it is important to update behavior modification strategies as evidence of effectiveness becomes available[54] (**Box 1**). Even efficacious techniques will be ineffective if they are too difficult or time consuming for the client to implement. Focusing efforts on easy-to-implement strategies may improve compliance. When counseled on separation anxiety prevention via brief preadoption sessions or generic written advice, owners showed excellent compliance with leaving

Table 3
Behavioral management strategies for separation anxiety and noise aversions

Behavior Management Strategies	Separation Anxiety	Noise Aversions
Avoidance	• Avoid leaving the dog home alone when possible • Avoid cues that predict departure • Avoid confinement if the dog does not tolerate it	• Avoid leaving the dog home alone during noise events • Avoid taking the dog outdoors during noise events • Avoid confinement if the dog does not tolerate it • Encourage the dog to rest in an interior, windowless room
Environmental modification	• Use a combination of white noise and music to decrease intensity of noises that may cause agitation (ie, neighbors returning home) • Establish a safe and comfortable resting area for the dog	• Use white noise, calming music, and consider soundproofing to decrease the intensity of noises • Establish a safe and comfortable resting area for the dog
Modifying interactions	• Keep departures and arrivals low key • Avoid direct interactions (play, training, walks) 15–30 min before departures • Do not punish	• Provide comfort (physical contact and speaking in calm tones) if this helps to soothe the dog • Do not punish
Behavior modification	• Provide a long-lasting interactive treat 5–10 min before departures • Relaxation training • Cue-response-reward	• Provide a long-lasting interactive treat during noise events • Follow any loud noises immediately with a small high-value food treat • Relaxation training • Cue-response-reward

---

Box 1
Complex versus simple behavior modification plans

Treatment protocols for separation anxiety in several texts recommend changing the predictive value of predeparture cues (ie, picking up keys, putting on shoes) by practicing these departure routines without leaving the house[14,19]; this exercise has been part of behavior modification protocols in several clinical trials for the treatment of separation anxiety.[23,24,42,55] This exercise uses the classical conditioning technique of extinction by presenting the conditioned stimulus for the dog's anxiety (departure cues) without presenting the unconditioned stimulus for the dog's anxiety (owner absence).[56] Extinction can diminish anxiety elicited by the conditioned stimulus; however, this may take many trials and may be difficult to practically implement if several owner activities have become conditioned stimuli for departures. This technique also has the potential to increase anxiety[19,57] and shows poor compliance,[53] possibly because of these challenges. In the author's practice, extinction of departure cues is rarely recommended in the treatment of separation anxiety.

Desensitization and counterconditioning to fear-eliciting triggers is a behavior modification technique used to treat a range of behavioral disorders.[58] The desensitization and counterconditioning procedure involves identifying all stimuli that elicit the fear response, arranging these stimuli on a gradient from lowest to highest intensity, and starting exposure sessions at the lowest stimulus intensity. The stimulus is paired with something that elicits an automatic positive emotional response, such as food (classical counterconditioning), or with a cue for an alternative behavior that is then reinforced (operant counterconditioning). The intensity of the stimulus is gradually increased during subsequent sessions.[58] Throughout this process, it is essential that the intensity of the stimulus is never presented at a level that elicits the fear response or sensitization to the stimulus, and worsening of the fear response rather than desensitization will occur. This technique is effective in the treatment of fear and anxiety, but application for the treatment of separation-related distress and noise aversions presents several practical challenges. The fear-eliciting triggers for separation anxiety may be elements of the owner's departure routine or an absence of any duration, and it can be difficult or impossible for many owners to completely avoid these triggers throughout the desensitization process. The fear-eliciting triggers for noise aversions, especially those related to thunderstorms, may be so complex that they are difficult to replicate during desensitization sessions.[38] These stimuli are often unpredictable and uncontrollable, so dogs may be exposed to the full intensity of the stimulus before desensitization is completed, further prolonging the process. In addition to these challenges, compliance is poor,[24,53] and these techniques may intensify the dog's fear and anxiety if used incorrectly (ie, the intensity of the stimuli are too rapidly increased beyond the dog's tolerance).[20]

Although there are no direct comparisons of behavior modification programs available, less complicated behavior modification plans that focus on creating consistent interactions between owners and their dogs, eliminating the use of punishment, and rewarding desired behaviors have successfully treated separation anxiety in combination with medical therapy.[9,25,59] These protocols may prove easiest to implement in the clinical setting.

---

their dog a food-filled toy before departures.[10,24] Other studies using direct consultation with a veterinarian reported that clients complied with recommendations not to punish their dogs for house soiling or destructive behavior[23,53,55]; however, when this advice was relayed in written form only, owners continued to punish their dogs in response to house soiling or destructive behaviors.[24] This finding highlights the need for direct veterinary-client communication that gives the client an opportunity to ask questions about recommendations. Direct consultation also provides the clinician opportunity to modify the treatment plan based on the client's needs and abilities.

Separation Anxiety

Avoidance

Avoidance, when possible, is critical in reducing the intensity of the dog's distress as well as preventing further injury, property destruction, noise complaints, fines, or eviction. Options include placing the dog in daycare, taking the dog to work, hiring a pet sitter, or having a friend stay with the dog. These options may not be available to some clients due to owner- or dog-related factors.

Environmental modification

The goal of environmental modification is to make the environment as peaceful and comfortable for the dog as possible. Options include using a combination of white noise and music to muffle sounds that may cause agitation (ie, neighbors returning home, traffic noises) Establishing a safe, comfortable, and secure resting area for the dog can help. This "safe space" may be a crate, closet, or other location the dog feels safe, but the dog should not be forced to remain in a crate or small room unless it is comfortable with confinement.[2,19]

Modifying interactions

Owners should keep departures and arrivals as low key as possible and avoid direct interactions—such as play, training, or walks—immediately before departures.[2] In addition, owners should not punish the dog verbally or physically for destruction or house soiling that occurs in their absence, because this will not prevent reoccurrence of unwanted behaviors and will escalate the dog's distress. Although compliance with this advice is generally good,[23,55] some owners may argue that these punishments are justified because the dog appears "guilty" when they return home, suggesting that the dog knows it did something wrong. Rather than an admission of guilt or knowledge of wrongdoing, "guilty-look" behaviors are signs of appeasement used to diffuse conflicts. A few studies have investigated the "guilty look" in dogs and demonstrate that dogs' appeasement behaviors are in response to the owner's body language and possibly the context in which punishment has previously been administered, not a response to the "forbidden" behaviors.[60,61]

Behavior modification

Behavior modification exercises focus on improving the dog's association with the owner's absence as well as teach the dog how to be relaxed:

- Provide a long-lasting interactive treat (eg, Kong filled with palatable food) 5 to 10 minutes before owner's departure. This treat may distract the dog from the owner's departure as well as improve its emotional state.[14]
- Reinforce relaxation may be achieved by reinforcing the dog with a small treat whenever it is observed relaxing in the owner's presence, ideally several feet away from the owner.[14,25] Alternatively, relaxation can be taught in regular short training sessions (**Box 2**).
- Use a cue-response-reward pattern of interactions to improve consistency and teach the dog a calm way to ask for everything. Dogs are asked to sit before any interaction, including petting, play, feeding, going outdoors, or coming indoors. The sit response is followed by food, petting, attention, or access to the desired consequence. This exercise teaches the dog that a simple behavior (sit) always results in a positive outcome and can decrease anxiety.[9,14,25]

Confinement Distress

Dogs with confinement distress may show minimal or no signs of distress when home alone and not confined. These dogs can be identified via video, and treatment may be as simple as leaving the dog loose when home alone. The owners can close off certain rooms or areas of the home to restrict the dog's access. Streaming live video is ideal

---

Box 2
Relaxation training step by step

This exercise uses the technique of shaping. Once the goal behavior is defined, training begins by reinforcing some behavior the dog already does that is an approximation to the goal and then gradually reinforcing behaviors that are successively closer to that goal.[62] In relaxation training, the trainer/owner will mark and reinforce the dog as he or she gets closer to lying in a relaxed posture on the mat. A marker is used to clearly communicate to the dog which behavior is reinforced.[62] Markers commonly used in dog training include specific words (ie, yes) or sounds (ie, clicker) that have been repeatedly paired with food.

Example training plan:

1. Place the training mat down
2. Mark/treat the dog for looking at or turning toward the mat. *For steps 2 to 7, toss the treat away from the mat so the dog has to return to the mat to get reinforced again.
3. Mark/treat the dog for any movement toward the mat.
4. Mark/treat the dog for placing a paw on the mat.
5. Mark/treat the dog for standing with all 4 paws on the mat.
6. Mark/treat the dog for sitting on the mat.
7. Mark/treat the dog for lying on the mat.
8. After the dog has learned to lie down on the mat, extend the time he or she stays down before the mark/treat. *Once the dog is approaching the mat and lying down consistently, transition to rewarding the dog *on the mat* to promote a relaxed position.
9. Mark/treat any relaxed behaviors, including head on paws or mat, hip rocked to one side, hind legs extending from body, rolling to one side.
10. If the dog gets stuck at any step, return to a previously successful step where it was reinforced frequently. Slowly introduce small steps toward the goal behavior.

Tips:

- Keep training sessions to 2 to 3 minutes.
- Remove the training mat between sessions.
- If there are 2 or more dogs in the house, train with each dog separately.
- Once the dog is consistently lying in a relaxed posture on the mat, move the mat to various locations around the house to teach the dog the mat may be available anywhere and he or she will always be rewarded for relaxing on it.

---

for evaluation if the dog has a history of destruction or escape behaviors so that the owner can monitor in real time and return immediately if signs of distress are observed. If the dog experiences a combination of confinement distress and separation anxiety, confinement to a cage or crate should be avoided and treatment of separation anxiety should be initiated.

Noise Aversions

Avoidance
Complete avoidance of noise triggers related to weather or fireworks is often impossible, but dogs should not be taken outdoors during storms or fireworks. Encouraging the dog to rest in an interior windowless room may reduce perceived noise intensity.

Environmental modification
The goal of environmental modification is to make the environment as peaceful and comfortable for the dog as possible during noise events. Acoustic tiles may be set up

in the dog's hiding space to soundproof the area, and black-out window coverings can be used to minimize the sight of flashing lights that may accompany fireworks or electrical storms. The intensity of outdoor sounds may be diminished by increasing the level of white noise in the house through use of white noise machines or fans, and increasing the level of noise in the home by playing music or TV. The use of music or TV should be based on the dog's tolerance, because some dogs may show fear in response to these stimuli.

Modifying interactions

Owners should be coached to avoid punishing the dog or forcing confinement because these methods will escalate the dog's distress. Opinions vary on whether to comfort dogs with noise aversions (**Box 3**).

Behavior modification

Behavior modification exercises focus on changing the dog's response to noise triggers as well as teaching the dog how to be relaxed.

- Providing a long-lasting interactive treat (eg, Kong filled with palatable food) during the noise event. This treat may distract the dog from the event as well as improve its emotional state.[14]
- Classical counterconditioning: In this exercise, the unpleasant stimulus (ie, thunder) is followed immediately by something that elicits a strong positive emotional response from the dog (ie, small piece of favored food). With regular practice, the dog learns that the loud noise predicts the pleasant event (food) and its fear and anxiety may diminish.[58]
- Reinforcing relaxation: This may be achieved by reinforcing the dog with a small treat whenever it is observed relaxing in the owner's presence. Alternatively, relaxation can be taught in scheduled training sessions (see **Box 2**).

Treatment Recommendations for Comorbidity

Patients presenting with a combination of separation anxiety, noise aversions, and/or confinement distress will benefit from the techniques described above in addition to the following:

Box 3
To comfort or not to comfort?

Opinions on whether to comfort frightened dogs vary among veterinary behaviorists,[2,21,39,63,64] and there are no controlled studies to evaluate the effectiveness or harm of comforting behaviors in the treatment of noise aversions. A survey of New Zealand pet owners showed that higher severity of noise fear was associated with owner-comforting behavior; however, a causal relationship cannot be made with this type of study, and it is possible that owners are more likely to comfort animals that show more intense signs of fear.[5] Another laboratory-based study investigated the behavioral and physiologic responses of beagles to a familiar person's 3 styles of greeting behaviors following a short absence. Results showed that dogs who were greeted with calm positive interactions, including physical touch, showed elevated levels of oxytocin even after the interaction ended and a more pronounced decrease in cortisol compared with dogs that were greeted verbally without physical touch and to dogs that were ignored upon reunion. These findings suggest that reciprocal physical contact between dogs and humans has beneficial calming effects,[65] although results cannot be directly extrapolated to companion dogs with behavioral disorders. Until more is known, whether to comfort a frightened dog should be based on the dog's response. If the dog appears comforted by owner attention, the owners can be encouraged to soothe their dog when distressed. If the dog does not appear comforted by these interactions, other behavior modification techniques should be attempted to assist the frightened dog.

- Avoid leaving the dog home alone during storms
- Avoid confining the dog when home alone or during storms
- Use rapidly acting anxiolytics with a longer duration of effect (ie, trazodone, clonazepam) if storms are predicted and the owners have to be out of the house

FOLLOW-UP

Regular communication via follow-up appointments, phone calls, and electronic methods should be scheduled based on individual patient and client needs as well as the severity and complexity of the issue. Regular follow-up communication is recommended for separation anxiety, confinement distress, and noise aversions to monitor response to treatment and make modifications as needed. The use of video and behavioral diaries can help the clinician and owner to objectively monitor treatment response and highlight where to focus treatment efforts.

Video Monitoring for Separation Anxiety

Monitoring dogs with separation anxiety via video when home alone in a range of conditions, such as during the owner's typical workday as well as off-routine departures (ie, evenings or weekend outings) or when the owner leaves the dog more than once in a 24-hour period, can provide objective information on the dog's progress and indicate areas that need further work. If a dog walker is used to taking the dog out during the owner's workday, video should include the dog walker's arrival and departure to ensure this event is not contributing to or escalating the dog's distress. Based on client videos in the author's practice, many dogs cope better when left alone undisturbed for several hours than when they have a "break" midday. Dogs may show signs of improvement first during the owner's routine absences and may be slower to improve during off-routine absences or when the owner leaves more than once per day.

TREATMENT ADJUSTMENTS

Treatment modifications may include trials with other anxiolytic medications as well as adjustments in the behavioral management plan. Some patients may need long-term treatment with psychopharmaceutical drugs. In these cases, physical examination and laboratory evaluations performed at 6- to 12-month intervals will help to monitor for changes in the dog's health status that may affect response to treatment and the prescribed medications. In addition, if a sudden or unexplained illness occurs while a patient is on a psychopharmaceutical drug, physical and laboratory evaluations should be pursued.[20]

SUMMARY

Separation anxiety, confinement distress, and noise phobias are welfare issues affecting many companion dogs. Despite their prevalence, clients may not recognize or report these issues, and many dogs go untreated. Clients should be asked about behavioral concerns at every veterinary visit to identify and address issues early. Although clinical signs are nonspecific and these disorders can be comorbid, a behavioral history and video can assist in accurate diagnosis. If clients report predeparture and postdeparture distress in the absence of destruction, vocalization, and house soiling, video of the pet while home alone should be gathered to rule in or rule out separation anxiety. Treatment of these conditions using a combination of psychopharmaceutical and behavior modification is recommended to improve welfare as quickly as possible.

REFERENCES

1. Tiira K, Sulkama S, Lohi H. Prevalence, comorbidity, and behavioral variation in canine anxiety. J Vet Behav 2016;16(C):36–44.
2. Sherman BL, Mills DS. Canine anxieties and phobias: an update on separation anxiety and noise aversions. Vet Clin North Am Small Anim Pract 2008;38(5):1081–106.
3. Bradshaw JWS, McPherson JA, Casey RA, et al. Aetiology of separation-related behaviour in domestic dogs. Vet Rec 2002;151(2):43–6.
4. Storengen LM, Lingaas F. Noise sensitivity in 17 dog breeds: prevalence, breed risk and correlation with fear in other situations. Appl Anim Behav Sci 2015;171:152–60.
5. Blackwell EJ, Bradshaw JWS, Casey RA. Fear responses to noises in domestic dogs: prevalence, risk factors and co-occurrence with other fear related behaviour. Appl Anim Behav Sci 2013;145(1–2):15–25.
6. Dale AR, Walker JK, Farnworth MJ, et al. A survey of owners' perceptions of fear of fireworks in a sample of dogs and cats in New Zealand. N Z Vet J 2010;58(6):286–91.
7. Overall KL, Dunham AE, Frank D. Frequency of nonspecific clinical signs in dogs with separation anxiety, thunderstorm phobia, and noise phobia, alone or in combination. J Am Vet Med Assoc 2001;219(4):467–73.
8. Flannigan G, Dodman NH. Risk factors and behaviors associated with separation anxiety in dogs. J Am Vet Med Assoc 2001;219(4):460–6.
9. Cannas S, Frank D, Minero M, et al. Video analysis of dogs suffering from anxiety when left home alone and treated with clomipramine. J Vet Behav 2014;9:50–7.
10. Herron ME, Lord LK, Husseini SE. Effects of preadoption counseling on the prevention of separation anxiety in newly adopted shelter dogs. J Vet Behav 2014;9(1):13–21.
11. Buller K, Ballantyne KC. Living with and loving a pet with behaviour problems: the impact on caregivers. In: Proceedings of the 11th International Veterinary Behaviour Meeting. Samorin, Slovakia. Wallingford, September 14–16, 2017. CABI. p. 128–9. https://doi.org/10.1079/9781786394583.0128.
12. Johnston E, Olson L. The neural substrates of fear and anxiety. In: The feeling brain: the biology and psychology of emotions. New York: W. W. Norton & Company; 2015. p. 65–98.
13. Ogata NN. Separation anxiety in dogs: what progress has been made in our understanding of the most common behavioral problems in dogs? J Vet Behav 2016;16(C):28–35.
14. Landsberg GM, Hunthausen W, Ackerman L. Fears, phobias, and anxiety disorders. In: Behavior problems of the dog and cat. 3rd edition. Saunders Limited; 2013. p. 181–210.
15. Herron ME, Shreyer T. The pet-friendly veterinary practice: a guide for practitioners. Vet Clin North Am Small Anim Pract 2014;44(3):451–81.
16. Frank D. Recognizing behavioral signs of pain and disease. Vet Clin North Am Small Anim Pract 2014;44(3):507–24.
17. Storengen LM, Boge SCK, Strøm SJ, et al. A descriptive study of 215 dogs diagnosed with separation anxiety. Appl Anim Behav Sci 2014;159:82–9.
18. Landsberg GM, Mougeot I, Kelly S, et al. Assessment of noise-induced fear and anxiety in dogs: modification by a novel fish hydrolysate supplemented diet. J Vet Behav 2015;10(5):391–8.

19. Horwitz DF. Separation-related problems in dogs and cats. In: Horwitz DF, Mills DS, editors. BSAVA manual of canine and feline behavioural medicine. 2nd edition. Gloucester (United Kingdom): British Small Animal Veterinary Association; 2010. p. 146–58.

20. Overall K. Abnormal canine behaviors and behavioral pathologies not primarily involving pathologic aggression. In: Manual of clinical behavioral medicine for dogs and cats. Elsevier Health Sciences; 2013. p. 231–311.

21. Palestrini C, Minero M, Cannas S, et al. Video analysis of dogs with separation-related behaviors. Appl Anim Behav Sci 2010;124(1–2):61–7.

22. Sherman BL, Landsberg GM, Reisner IR, et al. Effects of reconcile (fluoxetine) chewable tablets plus behavior management for canine separation anxiety. Vet Ther 2007;8(1):18–31.

23. King JN, Sherman BL, Overall KL, et al. Treatment of separation anxiety in dogs with clomipramine: results from a prospective, randomized, double-blind, placebo-controlled, parallel-group, multicenter clinical trial. Appl Anim Behav Sci 2000;67(4):255–75.

24. Blackwell EJ, Casey RA, Bradshaw JWS. Efficacy of written behavioral advice for separation-related behavior problems in dogs newly adopted from a rehoming center. J Vet Behav 2016;12(c):13–9.

25. Frank D. Animal behavior case of the month. J Am Vet Med Assoc 2005;227(6): 890–2.

26. Scaglia E, Cannas S, Minero M, et al. Video analysis of adult dogs when left home alone. J Vet Behav 2013;8(6):412–7.

27. Konok V, Dóka A, Miklósi Á. The behavior of the domestic dog (Canis familiaris) during separation from and reunion with the owner: a questionnaire and an experimental study. Appl Anim Behav Sci 2011;135(4):300–8.

28. Rehn T, Keeling LJ. The effect of time left alone at home on dog welfare. Appl Anim Behav Sci 2011;129(2–4):129–35.

29. Parthasarathy V, Crowell-Davis SL. Relationship between attachment to owners and separation anxiety in pet dogs (Canis lupus familiaris). J Vet Behav 2006; 1(3):109–20.

30. McGreevy PD, Masters AM. Risk factors for separation-related distress and feed-related aggression in dogs: additional findings from a survey of Australian dog owners. Appl Anim Behav Sci 2008;109(2–4):320–8.

31. Cannas S, Frank D, Minero M, et al. Puppy behavior when left home alone: changes during the first few months after adoption. J Vet Behav 2010;5(2): 94–100.

32. Irimajiri M, Crowell-Davis SL. Animal behavior case of the month. Separation anxiety. J Am Vet Med Assoc 2014;245(9):1007–9.

33. Overall KL, Dunham AE, Juarbe-Diaz SV. Phenotypic determination of noise reactivity in 3 breeds of working dogs: a cautionary tale of age, breed, behavioral assessment, and genetics. J Vet Behav 2016;16:113–25.

34. Levine E. Sound sensitivities. In: Horwitz DF, Mills DS, editors. BSAVA manual of canine and feline behavioural medicine. 2nd edition. Gloucester (United Kingdom): British Small Animal Veterinary Association; 2010. p. 159–68.

35. Mariti C, Raspanti E, Zilocchi M, et al. The assessment of dog welfare in the waiting room of a veterinary clinic. Anim Behav 2015;24(3):299–305.

36. Landsberg GM, Hunthausen W, Ackerman L. Is it behavioral, or is it medical?. In: Landsberg GM, Hunthausen W, Ackerman L, editors. Behavior problems of the dog and cat. 3rd edition. Saunders Limited; 2013. p. 75–94.

37. Overall KL. Medical differentials with potential behavioral manifestations. Vet Clin North Am Small Anim Pract 2003;33:213–29.
38. Crowell-Davis SL, Seibert L, Sung W, et al. Use of clomipramine, alprazolam, and behavior modification for treatment of storm phobia in dogs. J Am Vet Med Assoc 2003;222(6):744–8.
39. Sherman BL. Keynote presentation: use of psychopharmacology to reduce anxiety and fear in dogs and cats: a practical approach. In: Proceedings of the 11th International Veterinary Behaviour Meeting. Samorin, Slovakia, Wallingford, September 14–16, 2017. CABI. p. 9–19. https://doi.org/10.1079/9781786394583.0009.
40. Landsberg GM, Melese P, Sherman BL, et al. Effectiveness of fluoxetine chewable tablets in the treatment of canine separation anxiety. J Vet Behav 2008; 3(1):12–9.
41. Podberscek AL, Hsu Y, Serpell JA. Evaluation of clomipramine as an adjunct to behavioural therapy in the treatment of separation-related problems in dogs. Vet Rec 1999;145(13):365–9.
42. Karagiannis CI. Dogs with separation-related problems show a "less pessimistic" cognitive bias during treatment with fluoxetine (Reconcile™) and a behaviour modification plan. BMC Vet Res 2015;11(1):1–10.
43. Harding EJ, Paul ES, Mendl M. Animal behaviour: cognitive bias and affective state. Nature 2004;427(6972):312.
44. Mendl M, Burman OHP, Parker RMA, et al. Cognitive bias as an indicator of animal emotion and welfare: emerging evidence and underlying mechanisms. Appl Anim Behav Sci 2009;118(3–4):161–81.
45. Mendl M, Brooks J, Basse C, et al. Dogs showing separation-related behaviour exhibit a "pessimistic" cognitive bias. Curr Biol 2010;20(19):R839–40.
46. Gruen ME, Sherman BL. Use of trazodone as an adjunctive agent in the treatment of canine anxiety disorders: 56 cases (1995-2007). J Am Vet Med Assoc 2008; 233(12):1902–7.
47. Ogata NN, Dodman NH. The use of clonidine in the treatment of fear-based behavior problems in dogs: an open trial. J Vet Behav 2011;6(2):130–7.
48. Gruen ME, Roe SC, Griffith E, et al. Use of trazodone to facilitate postsurgical confinement in dogs. J Am Vet Med Assoc 2014;245(3):296–301.
49. Crowell-Davis SL, Murray T. Veterinary psychopharmacology. Blackwell Publishing; 2006. p. 1–270.
50. Fatjo J, Landsberg GM, Hunthausen W, et al. Pharmacologic intervention in behavioral therapy. In: Behavior problems of the dog and cat. 3rd edition. Saunders Limited; 2013. p. 113–38.
51. Korpivaara M, Laapas K, Huhtinen M, et al. Dexmedetomidine oromucosal gel for noise-associated acute anxiety and fear in dogs-a randomised, double-blind, placebo-controlled clinical study. Vet Rec 2017;180(14):356–7.
52. Ballantyne KC, Buller K. Experiences of veterinarians in clinical behavior practice: a mixed-methods study. J Vet Behav 2015;10(5):376–83.
53. Takeuchi Y, Houpt KA, Scarlett JM. Evaluation of treatments for separation anxiety in dogs. J Am Vet Med Assoc 2000;217(3):342–5.
54. Thielke LE, Udell MAR. The role of oxytocin in relationships between dogs and humans and potential applications for the treatment of separation anxiety in dogs. Biol Rev Camb Philos Soc 2017;92(1):378–88.
55. Blackwell EJ, Casey RA, Bradshaw JWS. Controlled trial of behavioural therapy for separation-related disorders in dogs. Vet Rec 2006;158(16):551–4.
56. Mazur JE. Basic principles of classical conditioning. In: Learning & behavior, 7th edition. New York: Routledge; 2016. p. 48–74.

57. Amat M, Camps T, Brech SL, et al. Separation anxiety in dogs: the implications of predictability and contextual fear for behavioural treatment. Anim Behav 2014; 23(3):263–6.

58. Landsberg GM, Hunthausen W, Ackerman L. Treatment-behavior modification techniques. In: Behavior problems of the dog and cat. 3rd edition. Saunders Limited; 2013. p. 95–112.

59. Seksel K. Two approaches to managing separation anxiety. In: Proceedings of the 11th International Veterinary Behaviour Meeting. Samorin, Slovakia, Wallingford, September 14–16, 2017. CABI. p. 92–3. https://doi.org/10.1079/9781786394583. 0092.

60. Horowitz A. Disambiguating the "guilty look": salient prompts to a familiar dog behaviour. Behav Processes 2009;81(3):447–52.

61. Hecht J, Miklósi Á, Gácsi M. Behavioral assessment and owner perceptions of behaviors associated with guilt in dogs. Appl Anim Behav Sci 2012;139(1–2): 134–42.

62. Pryor K, Ramirez K. Modern animal training: a transformative technology. In: McSweeney FK, Murphy ES, editors. The Wiley Blackwell handbook of operant and classical conditioning. John Wiley & Sons; 2014. p. 455–82.

63. Bennett SL. Noise aversion: comforting your pet. American Veterinarian; 2017. Available at: http://www.americanveterinarian.com/videos/noise-aversion-comforting-your-pet. Accessed October 15, 2017.

64. Hoffman J. A new treatment for dogs scared by thunder and fireworks. New York Times 2016. Available at: https://well.blogs.nytimes.com/2016/06/28/why-thunder-and-fireworks-make-dogs-anxious/. Accessed October 15, 2017.

65. Rehn T, Handlin L, Uvnäs-Moberg K, et al. Dogs' endocrine and behavioural responses at reunion are affected by how the human initiates contact. Physiol Behav 2013. https://doi.org/10.1016/j.physbeh.2013.10.009.

Managing Canine Aggression in the Home

Amy Pike, DVM

KEYWORDS

- Canine aggression • Treatment goals • Strategies • Management

KEY POINTS

- Canine aggression that occurs in the home can be a dangerous diagnosis with costly consequences to all members of the household.
- Management is a key modality in the treatment of canine aggression in the home.
- A thorough history will detail each trigger, target, and context and allow for the veterinary team to put together a comprehensive management plan.
- Management allows for the avoidance of future aggressive episodes and minimizes the risks associated with living with a patient with these diagnoses.
- Although risk cannot be mitigated 100%, thorough management can create a safe environment for the implementation of the behavior treatment plan.

INTRODUCTION

Canine aggression remains a serious problem in our society. It is the number 1 reason cited for relinquishment of dogs to shelters,[1,2] and according to the Centers for Disease Control and Prevention, there are approximately 4.5 million dog bites to humans each year in the United States.[3] When a dog is aggressive, owners may be struggling with the decision to keep it, rehome it, or euthanize it. Whenever an owner is faced with aggression, they should immediately seek advice from their veterinarian for several reasons. First and foremost, aggression, especially that which is sudden in onset, can be due to an underlying medical cause.[4] In addition, veterinarians are in the unique position of being the foremost expert on issues that impact both animal and human health, such as dog bites.

Unfortunately, like most diseases that veterinarians treat, there is no cure for aggression. If the owners decide they wish to keep the dog, management is going to be one of the hallmarks of treatment in order to prevent any further bite episodes. Management will decrease the risk associated with the aggression, stop the practice and perfection of the problematic behavior, and allow the implementation of an effective treatment plan. There are many types of aggression in the home that are very responsive to

The author has nothing to disclose.
Behavior Medicine Division, Veterinary Referral Center of Northern Virginia, Manassas, VA, USA
E-mail address: dramypike@vrc-nova.com

management, and management becomes especially important when there are at-risk age groups, such as young children,[5] immunocompromised, and the elderly.

HISTORY OF AGGRESSION IN THE HOME

There are many types of aggression that could manifest within the home. It is imperative that a thorough history of the aggressive episodes be taken, and diagnoses be determined before embarking on the management and treatment. A thorough history will help elucidate the triggers, the target, and the locations where the aggression occurs, which will then help the clinician delineate a specific management plan. It is also important that the clinician determine whether the aggression is offensive or defensive in nature. Offensive aggression is classified as aggression toward the victim without apparent interaction attempts by the victim. Defensive aggression is an attempt to increase the distance between the dog and the victim and occurs when the victim has attempted interaction with the dog. Although both defensive and offensive aggression are rooted in fear, offensive aggression can be much more dangerous to the target, leading to a much more rigid management plan that must be adhered to. Detailed instructions on history taking is covered in Elizabeth Stelow's article, "Diagnosing Behavior Problems: A Guide for Practitioners," in this issue, but clinicians can also adapt the SOCRATES method of pain assessment often used in human medicine[6] for a concise history of aggression which will determine the triggers, the targets, and the locations needed for the management plan.

S—site: Where does the aggression take place? Examples: Is it when the dog is on the bed, on the couch, in the kitchen, only in the backyard, and so forth. Also, who is the target of the aggression?

O—onset: When did the aggression begin? Was it sudden or gradual in onset? Were there early warning signs like fear in certain situations; was there a traumatic event that preceded the onset of the aggression?

C—character: What is the manifestation of the aggression: barking, snarling, growling, lunging, snapping, nipping, or biting? If nipping or biting, are there scratches, punctures, tears, or multiple bites? Also, what does the dog look like during the episodes? Specifically, paying attention to body position and postures that would help elucidate if it is offensive or defensive in nature: ears, eyes, mouth, tail, and so forth. Does the dog bite once, and then retreat, or continue to bite and hold until pulled off of the target?

R—radiation: Does the aggression then extend to other circumstances? Does the dog continue to be aggressive after the trigger or stimulus has been removed?

A—associations: Are there any other associations with the aggression? Examples: when the food bowl is present; when the other dog in the house approaches the owner; when the grandkids are over, and so forth.

T—time course/pattern: Is there any pattern to the aggression? Examples: Does it only occur at night, only after a prolonged absence of the owner, only when people are visiting the home, and so forth.

E—exacerbating or relieving factors: What has been done in an attempt to help with the aggression? Have there been other training methods used previously? Are there any medication, supplements, nutraceuticals, pheromones, or over-the-counter products that they have tried? What helps and what makes it worse?

S—severity: According to the owner, how severe is the aggression on a scale of 1 to 10? This rating can help the clinician gauge how realistic the owners are being about the actual severity of the aggression, and how close they are to potentially euthanizing or rehoming the dog.

AGGRESSION WITHIN THE HOME: DIAGNOSES

Once a thorough history has been taken, the clinician can determine the diagnosis. Although there are many different diagnostic terms used in behavioral medicine, for the sake of consistency in this article, the following is a list of diagnostic terminology that will be used, with a brief description of each type of aggression that occurs within the confines of the home (inside and within the home property). Diagnoses are listed in alphabetical order.

Conflict Aggression

Conflict aggression is barking, snarling, growling, lunging, snapping, nipping, and/or biting directed toward people who live in the home with the dog or who visit on a very regular basis (nanny, dog walker, and so forth). Aggression occurs when the human's intentions are in conflict with the dog's intentions. For example, the owner pets the dog when the dog does not want to be petted and instead merely wants to rest in proximity to the owner. Owner attempts to physically place dog into confinement when the dog is resistant.

Fear-Based Aggression Toward Children

Fear-based aggression toward children includes barking, snarling, growling, lunging, snapping, nipping, and/or biting directed toward children, both familiar and unfamiliar. Children include children from newborn to 18 years of age. Most children are bitten by dogs that they know.[5] Children under the age of 7 are bitten most often when they initiate the interaction with the dog when the dog is resting or eating, whereas most older children are bitten when active, outdoors, and not initiating interaction with the dogs.[5]

Fear-Based Aggression Toward Unfamiliar People

Fear-based aggression toward unfamiliar people includes barking, snarling, growling, lunging, snapping, nipping, and/or biting directed toward people who are considered unfamiliar to the dog. Unfamiliar people may include family members or friends of the owners to which the dog has yet to become familiar with, despite numerous visits.

Inter-Dog Aggression During Times of High Arousal

Inter-dog aggression during times of high arousal includes barking, snarling, growling, lunging, snapping, nipping and/or biting directed toward other resident dogs in the home during times that increase arousal. Examples include when the doorbell rings, when the owners arrive home, or when play escalates.

Inter-Dog Aggression over Resources

Inter-dog aggression over resources includes barking, snarling, growling, lunging, snapping, nipping, and/or biting directed toward other resident dogs in the home over the context of a resource. Resources include food, food and water bowls, toys, bones, rawhides, or other long-lasting treats, resting spots (dog beds or human furniture), access through doors and hallways, and human attention.[7]

Inter-Dog Aggression with No Apparent Trigger

Inter-dog aggression with no apparent trigger includes barking, snarling, growling, lunging, snapping, nipping, and/or biting directed toward other resident dogs in the home upon sight, smell, or hearing the other dog. No resources or other triggering stimuli are apparently involved.

Irritable Aggression

Irritable aggression includes barking, snarling, growling, lunging, snapping, nipping, and/or biting directed toward people who live in the home with the dog or who visit on a very regular basis (nanny, dog walker, and so forth) when the dog is not feeling well, whether from illness, pain, or exhaustion.

Predatory Aggression

Predatory aggression includes stalking, lunging, snapping, nipping, and/or biting directed toward small animals that live in the home, such as cats, rabbits, hamsters, and so forth. The goal is to injure and/or kill the smaller animal, but may or may not consume (potentially other dogs, too).

Redirected Aggression

Redirected aggression includes barking, snarling, growling, lunging, snapping, nipping, and/or biting directed toward people and other dogs who live in the home with the dog or who visit on a very regular basis (nanny, dog walker, and so forth) when the inciting stimulus is not the actual/eventual target of the aggression.

Resource Guarding Aggression

Resource guarding aggression includes barking, snarling, growling, lunging, snapping, nipping, and/or biting directed toward people who live in the home with the dog or who visit on a very regular basis (nanny, dog walker, and so forth) over a resource. Resources include food, food and water bowls, toys, bones, rawhides or other long-lasting treats, resting spots (dog beds or human furniture), stolen items (trash, and so forth), and another person.

Territorial Aggression

Territorial aggression includes barking, snarling, growling, lunging, snapping, nipping, and/or biting directed toward people and other dogs walking by the property. Territorial aggression can occur both inside at the windows and doors or outside through fences or across property boundaries.

MANAGEMENT AND TREATMENT GOALS

Management is the key first step in any comprehensive behavior treatment plan. The patient will need to stop practicing and perfecting the problematic behavior before any further behavior modification can occur. The goal of management is to eliminate any further aggression, but it can be nearly impossible to bring the risk down to zero, for several reasons. First, the patient may have learned that aggression works to keep a person or another dog away. Alternatively, they may have learned that lower levels of aggression, such as growling, barking, and snarling, do not work because either the dog has been punished in the past for this behavior, or it has not resulted in the intended consequence of keeping people and other dogs away. Second, even the best management can potentially fail, such as when someone accidentally opens the door or forgets to put the muzzle on, or simply gets lax on adhering to a strict management plan because everything has been going so well recently. It is imperative that the clinician talk openly and honestly with the owners about the risks they are undertaking in keeping an aggressive dog. Although management and avoidance can minimize this risk, if the owner is unable to live with *any* potential risk of further aggression, or if the clinician deems the risk as too high for this family to reasonably undertake, the owners need to consider rehoming or euthanasia as viable alternatives. Unfortunately, rehoming would only be considered an option if the severity of the aggression is minimal and a change in ownership and/or environment would be in the pet's best interest for treatment.

STRATEGIES FOR MANAGEMENT

The following are specific strategies for avoidance and management of canine aggression within the home as well as which diagnoses it is applicable to. Strategies are listed in alphabetical order.

Avoid Performing the Triggering Circumstance

If the aggression stems from a person doing something to the dog that elicits the aggression, this should be avoided. In other words, if the dog becomes aggressive when the client attempts to do X, Y, or Z, then they should avoid doing X, Y, and Z. Examples include petting, disturbing when resting, trimming the dogs nails, putting on their leash, taking away a stolen object, running by the dog, and so forth. Alternate means to accomplish specific tasks are addressed in later discussion.

Applicable diagnoses include fear-based aggression toward unfamiliar people, fear-based aggression toward children, conflict aggression, irritable aggression, and resource guarding aggression.

Avoiding Punishment

Punishment has been shown to increase fear, anxiety, arousal, and aggression and can put the user at risk for being the target of aggression.[8,9] The clients should discontinue use of all punishment and aversive training devices, including prong collars, pinch collars, choke collars, verbal scolding, spanking, swatting, throwing water balloons or bags of chains/coins, spraying the dog with a water bottle, electronic fence collars, bark collars, and remote shock or "stimulation" collars immediately.

Applicable diagnoses apply to ALL.

Breaking up a Fight Between Dogs

Breaking up a fight between 2 dogs can cause one or both to redirect to the people, other dogs in the vicinity, or worsen the injuries sustained in the process so caution must be exercised. First, use a loud noise to quickly distract both dogs in hopes that they instantly let go of each other. Blasting an air horn, banging pots and pans together, or dropping a heavy book on the floor are all good ideas. Having the owner yell or clap their hands loudly can work, but may have the unintentional effect of escalating the fight if the dogs are fighting over human attention. If the dogs are outdoors, the client can spray the dogs with the garden hose on full stream. Then, the client can grab the back legs of the offensive dog and wheelbarrow her back away from the other dog. If there are 2 people available, this is preferably done with each grabbing one of the dogs. The client can also use a baby gate, a large flat piece of heavy duty cardboard, a couch cushion, or a large plastic laundry basket to push in between the 2 dogs. Break sticks are available commercially and allow the user to pry the jaws of one dog off of the other but may not prevent redirected aggression toward the user from occurring. Once separated, keep the dogs confined away from one another using any of the confinement techniques listed in later discussion until each has sufficiently calmed down and been checked over for any wounds. The separation period may need to be as much as 48 to 72 hours for some dogs.

Applicable diagnoses include inter-dog aggression (all 3 types) and redirected aggression.

Confinement

Confinement of the aggressive dog or dogs can be accomplished by several different methods. It is important to confine the dog *before* the onset of aggression, not as a means of punishment after the aggression has occurred. Confinement will be easier to use as a technique when the triggering circumstances are predictable and discreet in nature.

Behind closed doors

Placing the dog in its own designated room can provide a safe means of separating it from the rest of the household. If there will be young children in the home, the door should either be locked with a key or combination that only an adult has, or a hook and eye latch installed at a level that is reachable only by an adult. Placing a warning sign on the door will also help people remember that the dog is being confined in there.

Baby gates

The style of baby gate needed will depend on the size of the entrance, the size of the dog, it's ability and/or willingness to push or jump over the gate, and what it is being confined away from. If the dog is being confined away from small children or other dogs, it may be necessary to employ 2 gates, whereby they are placed 2 to 3 feet apart from one another or in front of 2 separate confinement areas (one for each dog, or one for the dog and one where the children will be). If the dog is tall or can jump over the gate, it can be feasible to use 2 gates, one stacked on top of the other, to increase the vertical height of the confinement. The double-stacked gates also work if you are confining the dog away from cats in the household in order to prevent them from jumping over it into the confinement area.

Crate or kennel

Crates and kennels are excellent tools for confinement purposes (**Fig. 1**). The dog will need to be conditioned to go in willingly using high value food as a lure and for positive reinforcement training. Proper conditioning may take weeks for some dogs depending on their history with these tools. On average, most dogs will take longer to condition to a crate than they would to going into a room or behind a baby gate. There are numerous styles of crates available, including wire, hard-sided plastic, and soft-sided kennels. Although seemingly more flimsy, the soft-sided kennels may provide more protection for children in the home as there is no way for them to stick their hands through, thus further preventing bites from the dog. Crates should additionally

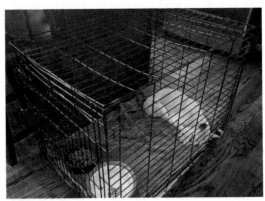

Fig. 1. Confinement in a crate. (*Courtesy of* Amy Pike, DACVB, Manassas, VA.)

be placed in locations where they will be inaccessible by the target of the aggression, and in a quiet area that allows the dog to relax and rest. The dog should be kept occupied with its favorite toys, and long-lasting treats such as a frozen stuffed Kong.

Exercise pens or playpens
If the dog is smaller and cannot jump over the edges, an exercise pen or human playpen can be used for confinement purposes. Because many do not have actual entrances that the dog can walk in and out of, the dog cannot be aggressive when picked up and handled because it will need to be picked up to go into and get out of the pen. Therefore, this would not be an appropriate means of confinement for conflict aggression.

Tethering indoors
Wall-mounted hooks can be used to tether the dog via a leash to a specific location in the home (**Fig. 2**). The hook would need to be securely mounted using the wall studs and located in an area where the dog would be unable to access people or other pets in the home (**Fig. 3**). Tethering does not, however, prevent people or other pets from encroaching on the area where the dog is located so this would not be an appropriate method in a home with young children or other pets that will not stay away from the aggressive dog.

Applicable diagnoses include ALL, except where otherwise noted.

Consent to Pet

People can be bitten when they pet a dog who either does not tolerate or enjoy petting, or who does not wish to be petted at that moment. Many dogs will approach people wanting to sniff, explore, or maintain proximity to the person, but they do not actually want to be petted. This approach is wrongly interpreted by the human as a desire to be petted, and the dog may become aggressive as a means to say "stop." Many trainers and behaviorists[10,11] espouse a "consent to pet" test as a means of literally asking the dog if petting is what they desire. A quick scratch underneath the chin or on the front of the chest is performed, and then the human stops and awaits the answer from the dog. If "yes," petting can proceed. If "no," petting must stop. **Table 1** provides indications of body postures and signs that indicate a yes and no answer.

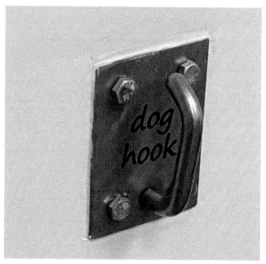

Fig. 2. Example of a wall hook used to tether a dog. (*Courtesy of* Amy Pike, DACVB, Manassas, VA.)

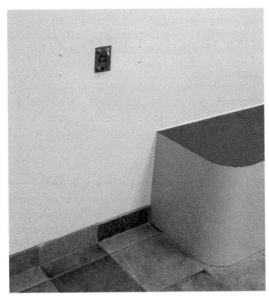

Fig. 3. Example of where a wall hook should be placed in the home. (*Courtesy of* Amy Pike, DACVB, Manassas, VA.)

For a video demonstration of the consent to pet test, visit the following sites:

https://www.youtube.com/watch?v=E09nsCe4lyQ- Yes, please!
https://www.youtube.com/watch?v=W88a-1MPr4g- No, thank you!

Applicable diagnoses include conflict aggression, fear-based aggression toward unfamiliar people, fear-based aggression toward children, and irritable aggression.

Control in the Yard

Fencing

Dogs that are held in the backyard of the home via tethering or behind an electronic fence can still become aggressive toward people and other dogs who enter the

Table 1
Consent to pet test

Body Part or Position	"Yes, Please!"—Dog Wants to Be Petted	"No, Thank You"—Dog Does Not Wish to Be Petted
Proximity to the person	Put their head or other part of their body near the person's hand	Lean away from the person; walk away; turn head away from the reaching hand
Feet	Paws at the person repeatedly	Raise one front paw off the ground, held tight to body
Mouth	Relaxed face and lips; tongue may loll	Tense face; lick their lips; yawn; snarling; growling
Eyes	Eyes are soft, droopy	Look away; show "whale eye" (whites of eyes showing at one corner); rapid eyelid blinking
Body	Loose, potentially wiggly	Generally stiff; may perform a "micro-freeze"
Other	Nudges at person's hand repeatedly	Displacement behaviors (scratching, licking, and so forth)

property because there is no physical prevention keeping others away. Tethering in the yard still has a high incidence of potential aggression[5] and is therefore not advisable. Because of easier installation, electronic fencing often encompasses both the front and back yards, which can put people and dogs walking, biking, or even driving by and up to the house at risk for aggression. Delivery personnel may attempt to drop off a package on the front step without knowing that the dog is outside before it is too late. Ideally, fencing should be privacy in nature, to prevent people and children from being able to stick their hands through the slats and dogs sticking paws or muzzles through. The fencing should be high enough to prevent the dog from jumping over and escaping into the neighborhood (5–6 feet high ideally). Key or combination locks should be used on the gates to ensure access to the yard only by those people who are entrusted with the key or code. Although not releasing the owners from liability associated with an incident, "Beware of Dog" signs can also be helpful to warn people of the potential for danger associated with entering the yard.

Supervision
If the owners are unwilling or unable to fence in their yard because of cost or neighborhood ordinances, then the owner must commit to only allowing the dog outside when it is leashed to, and properly supervised by, a responsible adult.

Drag Lines

Dogs with aggression may need to be quickly removed from any situation that puts them in danger of an altercation. However, if the dog will not respond to, or has not been taught, cues to move, physical manipulation may be necessary, which then puts the person in danger of aggression redirected toward them. The dog can wear a comfortable body harness with a 4- to 6-foot braided drag line attached to it, which can be grabbed at a safe distance away from the dog to then move them into a confinement location.
   Applicable diagnoses include ALL.

Escape Provisions for Other Pets

- Baby gates: Baby gates with small cutouts or doors in the gate can be useful for allowing cats to go through while keeping dogs out (**Figs. 4** and **5**).
- Microchip-activated pet doors: These doors can be a useful tool so a smaller pet, most often a cat, can escape into a room that is maintained as their own individual territory. Microchip-activated doors, such as the PetSafe Electronic Smart-Door (Radio Systems Corporation, Knoxville [TN]) or the SureFlap Microchip Pet Door (Sure Petcare, Clearwater [FL]), ensure that only the animal with the associated RFID chip can enter or exit through that door.
- Vertical spacing: Providing cats with additional vertical territory allows them to escape to higher ground away from a pursuing dog. They additionally provide resting spots away from other pets in the household. Cat trees, shelving, and even high furniture can increase the vertical spacing available to the cat. Owners must ensure that vertical spaces have multiple exit routes so that the cat does not become trapped at the top.

Applicable diagnoses include predatory aggression.

Managing Resources

Resources can be a major source of conflict and include food, empty food bowls, toys, bones, rawhides or other long-lasting treats, resting spots (dog beds or human furniture), stolen items (trash, and so forth), and a person. Dogs may guard their resources from other dogs in the household, other pets, children, or other adults.

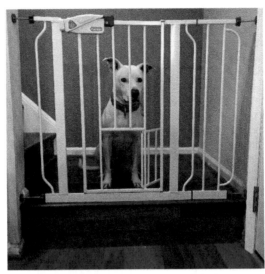

Fig. 4. Dog confined behind a baby gate. (*Courtesy of* Bethany Poese, Canine Lifestyle Academy.)

Toys, bones, rawhides and long-lasting food items

All items, such as toys, bones, rawhides and long-lasting food items, should be put out of visual and physical access of the dog. When a responsible adult determines it is time to allow the pet a resource, the pet must be confined away from people and other pets (see "Confinement" for options) before allowing the pet to have it. Ensure that long-lasting food items and bones are of a size that will be consumed in one setting and not something that will need to be removed from the dog before full consumption.

Food and empty food bowls

Feed the dog confined out of visual and physical access from other dogs and humans in the home (see "Confinement" for options). If the dog guards the container or closet where the food is stored, the dog must be placed into confinement before preparing food. Once the dog is finished and the food bowl is empty, the dog can be let out of confinement, but the bowl should not be picked up and removed until the dog is

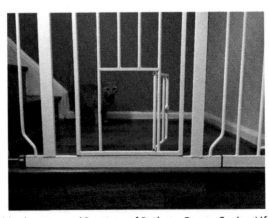

Fig. 5. Cat-accessible door open. (*Courtesy of* Bethany Poese, Canine Lifestyle Academy.)

sequestered in another location in the home, or placed in the backyard. Food bowls should be stored out of visual and physical access from the dog.

Resting spots

The dog should no longer be allowed to rest on human furniture if this is a resource of conflict. The dog can be taught to get off furniture using a cue such as "off" and rewarded for complying with a valuable treat. At no point should the dog ever be physically removed from the furniture, by grabbing the dog's collar or pushing the dog off, as these activities can lead to aggression and injury. An alternate resting spot, such as a dog bed or crate, can be provided and the dog taught to go there on cue and intermittently rewarded for lying down and staying there. If the dog is aggressive when resting on a dog bed, their use should be avoided. A crate or exercise pen can work as an alternative location.

Stolen objects

If the dog is prone to stealing things off countertops, care should be taken to keep items out of their reach on the counters. Place kitchen items on top of the refrigerator or inside the oven or microwave. Trash cans should be placed inside cabinets or closets. Alternatively, trash cans with a top lid that opens by stepping on a foot pedal can be used for dogs too small to tip them over. Techniques for retrieving stolen items are discussed later in "Retrieving stolen objects."

A person

If the dog guards a particular person from other pets, or even from other people, in the household, this person must not show the dog any attention or affection, or allow the dog on their lap whenever there are any other dogs or people in the vicinity. All attention can be given whenever the dog is confined away from others in the household.

Applicable diagnoses include inter-dog aggression over resources and resource guarding aggression.

Muzzles

Muzzles are an excellent tool to prevent injury toward people and other dogs. Basket muzzles are the preferred style of muzzle to use (indicated by red stars in **Fig. 6**) so the dog can still pant, drink water, and take treats while wearing it. The dog must be taught to wear the muzzle in a positive fashion, which can be done either by smearing a high

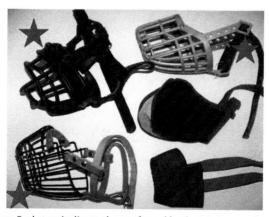

Fig. 6. Muzzle types. Red stars indicate the preferred basket style muzzles. (*Courtesy of* Amy Pike, DACVB, Manassas, VA.)

value food like peanut butter or liverwurst inside the muzzle (luring) and/or through shaping the dog to willingly stick their own nose into it.

A video example can be found at https://www.youtube.com/watch?v=wZN0H3FQr1A.

The muzzle must never be used as a punishment tool for showing aggressive behavior, only as a management tool before any possibility of aggression. One added benefit of using a muzzle on a dog is the potential that people and other owners may actually avoid crossing paths with you, thus making management in busy areas easier.[12] It is important to remember that making a dog safer with a muzzle does not give permission to then put them in an uncomfortable or aggression-provoking situation if it is unnecessary and otherwise manageable.

Applicable diagnoses include ALL.

Removing Visual Access to Outside the Home

In order to prevent any aggressive displays inside the home toward people or dogs going by outside of the house, there are several techniques.

- Keep solid front doors closed versus allowing storm or screen doors to be accessible (as in **Fig. 7**).
- Remove resting spots where dogs perch to watch out the window. Many owners have benches or furniture that can be pulled away from the window so the dogs no longer sit in wait for people/dogs going by the house.
- Close any window blinds or curtains. This only works if the dog will not push aside the blockade. Plantation shutters (**Fig. 8**) may be the most resilient.
- Use cardboard or construction paper affixed to the outside of the windows to temporarily block visual access.

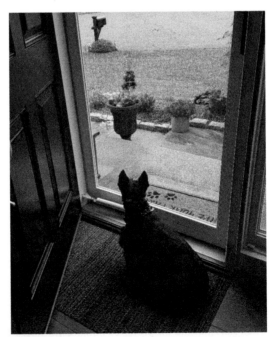

Fig. 7. Dog looking out glass door. (*Courtesy of* Amy Pike, DACVB, Manassas, VA.)

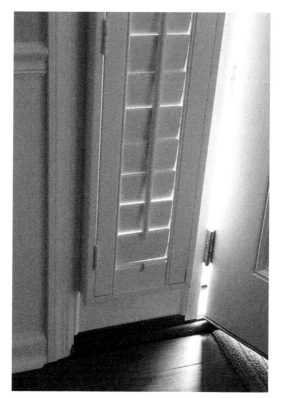

Fig. 8. Plantation shutters covering windows. (*Courtesy of* Amy Pike, DACVB, Manassas, VA.)

- Apply frosted window film from a home improvement store to limit visual access while still letting light through the window or glass door (**Fig. 9**).

Applicable diagnoses include inter-dog aggression during times of high arousal, redirected aggression, territorial aggression, and fear-based aggression toward unfamiliar people.

Retrieving a Stolen Object

When a dog obtains something that they should not have or that is potentially dangerous or toxic, there are several techniques that can be used to retrieve the object that will not elicit aggression. The first thing to remember is to not chase the dog around or just reach into their mouth in an attempt to grab the object as both of these methods can result in aggression or even cause the dog to swallow the object faster in an effort to keep it away from the person.

Distraction

Dogs will often drop something in their possession to go investigate something that peaks their interest even more. Options of distraction include ringing the doorbell, getting the dog's leash and asking them to go for a walk, opening the refrigerator door and getting their favorite human food item out, or opening the back door and asking them if they want to go outside. If there are 2 people in the house, once the dog has left the inappropriate object behind to investigate the distractor, the other

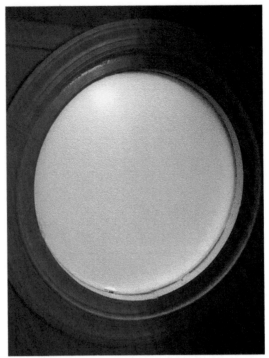

Fig. 9. Frosted window film allows light in but limits visual access. (*Courtesy of* Amy Pike, DACVB, Manassas, VA.)

person can then go retrieve it. If there is only one person available, once the dog is sufficiently distracted from the object, place the dog in confinement before retrieving the stolen object.

Trade
Dogs should be taught to trade on cue, and positively rewarded for compliance, as part of initial obedience training. However, even if the dog has not yet been taught to trade, or it is still a work in progress, most dogs will gladly spit out what has been stolen for a moderately large quantity of a very high value food, such as a hot dog or string cheese. If the dog grabs an object, someone can immediately go to the refrigerator to get the already prepared and stored high value food item, bring it to the dog and put it right up to their nose. Once the dog drops the object and starts to eat the food item out of the presenting hand, the person can then quickly grab the object with their other hand and place it behind their back or in their pocket. This method of retrieval takes proper prior planning so that the high value food item is always kept in stock and is ready to go at a moment's notice. This method should NOT be used for dogs with resource guarding aggression so intense that they cannot be fed directly from your hand and with those who will not allow someone to grab the object once it has been dropped. If the dog cannot eat from the hand, but is still motivated by the high value food, the food can be shown to the dog and then tossed 4 to 5 feet away from the person in order to also move the dog a safe distance away from them and the object.

Applicable diagnoses include resource guarding aggression.

Reevaluation, Readjustment, Recurrence

Clinicians should plan to follow up frequently and on a regular basis in cases of aggression. The clients will need support and guidance in implementing the management plan. In addition, they may feel frustrated and overwhelmed with the amount of changes needed in their household in order to prevent any further aggression. Through diligent follow-up, it may come to light that the initial management plan did not completely address the triggers or was inevitably too difficult for the clients to implement and the management plan will need to be revised. Nurses and assistants can be used for follow-up and trained to take a follow-up history asking about any new incidences or difficulty implementing the plan. Follow-up could be via e-mail, via telephone, or in the office.

Despite a thorough history at the time of presentation, future episodes of aggression may occur. It is important to remember that management can fail. Human error or relaxation of protocols can lead to detrimental consequences, and owners must be vigilant in order for management to succeed. In addition, as the patient matures, there may also be new incidences of aggression whose triggers or scenarios were not previously identified. New incidences can be the result of new or worsening fears and anxieties from traumatic events or learned associations. Clinicians must convey this potential to owners so that owners will not feel they have failed in implementation of the management plan nor that this is an indication of a worsening prognosis for this pet. Furthermore, if owners see the recent incidences of aggression as a failure of the initial plan in managing the aggression, they may seek additional help elsewhere.

SUMMARY

Canine aggression that occurs in the home can be a dangerous diagnosis with costly consequences to all members of the household. Management is a key modality in the treatment of canine aggression in the home. A thorough history will detail each trigger, target, and context and allow for the veterinary team to put together a comprehensive management plan. Management allows for the avoidance of future aggressive episodes and minimizes the risks associated with living with a patient with these diagnoses. Although risk cannot be mitigated 100%, thorough management can create a safe environment for the implementation of the behavior treatment plan.

REFERENCES

1. Kwan JY, Bain MJ. Owner attachment and problem behaviors related to relinquishment and training techniques of dogs. J Appl Anim Welf Sci 2013;16(2):168–83.
2. Salman MD, New JG Jr, Scarlett JM, et al. Human and animal factors related to relinquishment of dogs and cats in 12 selected animal shelters in the United States. J Appl Anim Welf Sci 1998;1(3):207–26.
3. Available at: https://www.cdc.gov/features/dog-bite-prevention/index.html. Accessed September 15, 2017.
4. Overall KL. Medical differentials with potential behavioral manifestations. Vet Clin North Am Small Anim Pract 2003;33(2):213–29.
5. Reisner IR, Nance ML, Zeller JS, et al. Behavioral characteristics associated with dog bites to children presenting to an urban trauma center. Inj Prev 2011;17(5):348–53.
6. Briggs E. Assessment and expression of pain. Nurs Stand 2010;25(2):35–8.
7. Wrubel KM, Moon-Fanelli AA, Maranda LS, et al. Interdog household aggression: 38 cases (2006–2007). J Am Vet Med Assoc 2011;238(6):731–40.

8. Herron ME, Shofer FS, Reisner IR. Survey of the use and outcome of confrontational and non-confrontational training methods in client-owned dogs showing undesired behaviors. Appl Anim Behav Sci 2009;117(1):47–54.

9. Hiby EF, Rooney NJ, Bradshaw JW. Dog training methods: their use, effectiveness and interaction with behavior and welfare. Anim Welf 2004;13(1):63–70.

10. Available at: https://ppgworldservices.com/2016/10/13/does-your-dog-really-want-to-be-petted-2/. Accessed September 21, 2017.

11. Donaldson J. Oh behave!: dogs from Pavlov to Premack to Pinker. Dogwise Publishing; 2008.

12. Mariti C, Papi F, Zilocchi M, et al. Dog appeal to people: does it depend on dog features? European Veterinary Behavior Meeting. Hamburg, Germany, September 24–26, 2010. p. 55–6.

Vertical or Horizontal? Diagnosing and Treating Cats Who Urinate Outside the Box

Leticia Mattos de Souza Dantas, DVM, MS, PhD*

KEYWORDS

- Cat • Elimination • House soiling • Urine marking • Inappropriate elimination
- Feline idiopathic cystitis

KEY POINTS

- Feline elimination problems are often responsible for the relinquishment, abandonment, and euthanasia. Veterinarians might misdiagnose patients owing to cat individual variation and cases that are multifactorial.
- The main diagnostic umbrellas for elimination outside of the litter box are medical problems, toileting behavior outside of the litter box, and urine marking.
- Feline idiopathic cystitis is a common etiology either alone or in combination with other medical and behavioral problems.
- Treatment involves optimum litter box management, fulfilling cats' environmental needs, stress reduction and behavior therapy techniques, trigger removal, and medical management of underlying anxiety.

INTRODUCTION

Cats that urinate outside of their litter boxes are commonly presented to general practitioners, veterinary behaviorists, and other specialists in veterinary medicine. Clients search for information online, and spend a good amount of resources purchasing top-of-the-line litters and pet products that promise to make the problem disappear with no avail. Inappropriate elimination continues to be one of the most common problem behaviors in cats and causes millions of felines to be relinquished to shelters, abandoned to their own luck, and euthanized.[1–4] This article aims to present succinct and straightforward scientific information that will help veterinarians more easily

Disclosure Statement: The author has nothing to disclose.
Behavioral Medicine Service, University of Georgia Veterinary Teaching Hospital, University of Georgia College of Veterinary Medicine, 501 D.W. Brooks Drive, Athens, GA 30602, USA
* 1291 Willowynd Way, Watkinsville, GA 30677.
E-mail address: leticia.zoopsych@gmail.com

diagnose and treat a problem that can be as simple as a medical condition and as complex as multiple associated etiologies.[5]

FIRST THINGS FIRST: TERMINOLOGY AND INTRODUCTION TO DIFFERENTIAL DIAGNOSES

The first root of confusion for veterinarians when dealing with cats eliminating outside of their litter boxes is the misleading terminology found in multiple sources. Inappropriate elimination, a term commonly found in the scientific literature and lay publications, only means that the cat is failing to urinate in the litter box or previous designated or learned location.[6] Similarly, the term house soiling is also used to refer to the deposition of urine (or feces) on objects or vertical or horizontal surfaces in locations considered unacceptable to owners.[7] These are not diagnoses or an indication of a particular etiology. However, inappropriate elimination is frequently used to refer to the act of practicing toileting behavior outside of the litter box (therefore referring to physiologic micturition and not marking behavior), which adds to the confusion.[8]

In short, there are 3 main diagnostic umbrellas that need to be considered[5]:

- Medical problems,
- Toileting behavior (micturition) outside of the litter box, and
- Urine marking.

In theory, any medical problem that causes pain or discomfort (in any system of the body) and/or increases urgency, frequency, or leads to pain during urination can cause a cat to eliminate outside of the litter box. Common examples are diseases of the urinary tract, and endocrine, gastrointestinal, metabolic, and orthopedic disorders. Only after medical causes are excluded should behavioral diagnoses be considered.[5] Multifactorial cases (that involve medical problems in addition to behavioral or mental health causes) are not rare.[9]

Using a sandy substrate to eliminate and the toileting sequence itself are hardwired in the cat and very well-conditioned behaviors in kittenhood.[10] It is safe to assume that there is always a problem of some kind when a cat stops using their box. Cats will not do this to make the owners upset, out of spite, or to make a point. Marking behavior is complex, but a normal part of the cat's behavioral repertoire.[11,12] However, acute and chronic stress can be responsible.[5] A medical investigation is always the starting point.

Elimination of and marking with feces (middening) will not be reviewed in this article. Please consult Overall (2013)[13] for detailed information.

PHYSICAL EXAMINATION AND DIAGNOSTICS

Owing to the wide range of medical problems causing cats to miss the litter box (and the fact that mental health and behavioral disorders are diagnoses of exclusion in veterinary medicine), it is important to first examine the cat and take its medical history. Screening laboratory work such as complete blood count, serum biochemistry, urinalysis, and urine culture are considered to be the minimum workup.[5,9] The veterinary literature also recommends imaging studies of the abdomen and urinary tract.[14] Additional diagnostic tests will depend on the cat's history, physical examination, and initial laboratory findings.

PATIENT BEHAVIORAL HISTORY

The cat's history is a very important source of diagnostic information where elimination problems are concerned.[5] Many clients will not be open to paying for diagnostic tests and the primary care veterinarian is often limited to the clues given with the patient history to differentiate between the main diagnoses that can be involved in each case. It is important to keep in mind that some feline patients suffering from the some of the most common medical causes of elimination outside of the box (such as feline idiopathic cystitis [FIC] and musculoskeletal or joint disease) might have normal laboratory work and a normal physical examination.[14,15] The behavioral signs can the most revealing findings. The American Association of Feline Practitioners and International Society of Feline Medicine Guidelines for Diagnosing and Solving House-Soiling Behavior in Cats[9] includes a comprehensive history form that can be used by practitioners. A house plan or map is important to help the practitioner detect special patterns with the cat's elimination habits.

Important History Findings to Consider

Toileting behavior

When cats present with toileting behavior outside of their boxes, the elimination behavior still presents the same function, similar characteristics, and morphology of the elimination behavior of a normal cat.[5,9,16]

A few important points to be considered are as follows.

- Cats tend to be private when they eliminate. Cats with abnormal toileting behavior will often eliminate right next to their litter boxes or in a location of the house that is either hidden or has fewer people or less animal traffic (such as behind couches, bathrooms, bedrooms, closets, baskets, etc).
- Cats prefer substrates that quickly absorb urine (rugs, carpet, piles or baskets of clothes, pillows, drains, sinks, vases, etc). It is not uncommon that the client has never seen the cat eliminate and there could be confusion as to which cat is responsible (in a multicat household).
- Keeping the function of toileting behavior in mind, the puddles and stains of urine found are similar in volume to what would be seen in the litter box.
- When the behavior is witnessed, the cat presents a similar sequence typical of normal toileting behavior (digging, sniffing, circling, covering, and eliminating in a squatting position). Some cats act distressed (which can be a sign of pain and/or stress or anxiety) and the behavioral sequence might be incomplete when compared with a normal cat. Urine is typically voided in a horizontal surface. Not covering urine and/or feces is normal for many cats and it is not an indicator of a problem. A change from previous routine behavior, however (eg, when a cat that consistently used to cover their elimination suddenly starts rushing out of the box once it is finished urinating or defecating), can be indicative of issues.[16]
- The frequency can also mirror how often a cat normally urinates in a day (2–4 times). That piece of information might not be reliable when the reason for missing the litter box is a medical problem, however.
- Depending on the etiology or overriding cause of the problem, some cats will continue to use the litter box intermittently, whereas others will completely stop using it for urination, others will stop using it for urination and defecation, and other cats will have periods of normal behavior (using the litter box consistently) and periods of urinating in an alternative location.

Marking behavior

Urine marking significantly differs from toileting behavior starting with its function.[5,9,17,18]

- Being part of the feline's social behavior and communication repertoire, marking tends to happen in locations that meet 2 criteria: somewhere the urine spot can be easily seen and smelled by people and other animals, and some part of the cat's core environment and travel route within the house. Corners of furniture, windows, doorways, stairways and cat flaps are commonly preferred. Objects that emit heat (such as toasters or stoves, or electronic devices) and items newly introduced to the house or that carry new or concentrated scent (such as suitcases, new furniture, shoes, purses, and laundry baskets) are other frequently reported targets. Cats tend to urinate repeatedly on the same locations or items. Cats that mark windows are probably responding to a perceived threat or stressor outside of the house.
- Because the goal of marking the environment is not micturition, the amount of urine voided tends to be less compared with cats missing the box to toilet (provided that the cat does not have polyuria).
- In neutered or spayed cats, marking is usually triggered by stress and identifying the cause or causes is fundamental for controlling and preventing the problem. Social and/or territorial stress (either related to living in a multicat household with conflict or the presence of cats outside) and management changes (owner travel, changes in the family unit and routine) are frequent causes. Urine marking is common and expected in cats that are sexually intact.
- The frequency of occurrences will vary depending on what is leading the cat to mark and it does not correspond with micturition. Cats that have to deal with stray cats outside or internal feline conflict within the house might urine mark every day. Cats that mark in response to episodic triggers such as their owners traveling tend to urine mark occasionally.
- Cats typically mark with urine by spraying in a standing position, backing up to the location where urine will be voided on, with tail up and quivering, with an arched back. Some cats also tread on their feet. This posture will frequently lead to stains or urine spots that are found vertically or dripping. Cats usually will not approach the voided urine to dig, sniff or attempt to cover and might rush out as soon as they are done. Some cats mark in a squatting position, so all pieces of information provided by the patient history should be considered.
- Most cats that present with urine marking as their only elimination problem continue to use their litter box for micturition and defecation. When that is not observed (and findings listed on the section Toileting behavior are also observed), the veterinarian is likely dealing with a multifactorial case. Substrate preference is typically not seen when cats mark with urine.
- It is common that someone in the household has seen the cat mark.
- In multicat households, it is likely that more than one cat is marking. In fact, living in a multicat household is a risk factor for urine marking.
- Both males and females (regardless of their reproductive status) can urine mark.
- Cat with either confident or shy temperament can urine mark.

DIAGNOSES AND ETIOLOGIES
Medical Problems

Medical problems are often the primary reason causing cats to urinate outside of their litter boxes. As stated, any conditions that cause pain, discomfort of any kind, and/or an increase urine production, urgency, and frequency to urinate can be responsible. Experiencing pain and discomfort while using the litter box might lead to secondary learning processes of litter box aversion and a new location and/or subtract prefer-ence, making the problem more complex. Owing to this factor, resolution of the orig-inal medical condition does not necessarily lead to the cat going back to using the litter box. This is common example of a multifactorial case.[5–9]

FIC is among the leading causes associated with cats urinating outside of their litter boxes. It can be challenging for veterinarians because it is a diagnosis of exclusion, and not every client will be able to afford what the literature recommends for ruling out all other urinary tract conditions. In addition, cats with FIC often have a normal physical examination and laboratory work with no or mild abnormalities and there is no specific diagnostic test that can confirm it. However, the patient history can be really helpful. Cats with FIC not only might miss the litter box (periuria), but can also present intermittent signs of dysuria, pollakiuria, hematuria, overgrooming, and other general signs of increased stress. The problem might seem to resolve itself temporarily only to relapse again and it is commonly a chronic condition. Clients can often trace the first episode (and many times flare ups) to stressors or changes in management or in the cat's routine.[14,19–21]

Toileting or Elimination Outside of the Litter Box

There are a number of possible reasons that might lead a cat to stop using their litter boxes. Problems with the litter boxes' hygiene and management, social problems be-tween cats, and other stressors are common causes.[9]

Once again, information obtained by a detailed history will help the veterinarian to make the correct diagnosis. Using the litter box right after cleaning, avoiding touching the litter or the bottom of the box (some cats will try to eliminate balancing themselves on the edges of the box or will have 2 limbs inside and 2 outside of the box), rushing out of the box, and completing their behavioral sequence outside (such as digging on the floor next to the box) are all behaviors indicative of a cat who is bothered by some-thing that has to do with the litter box.[5]

Similar to urine marking, living in multicat house hold also puts cats at a higher risk for presenting toileting problems. Owing to the biology of their social behavior (using several types of marking behaviors to communicate and avoiding conflict when possible), social problems between cats can be missed by clients and remain unre-ported. Many clients, however, witness agonistic and avoidance behaviors between their cats and do not realize these behaviors can be related to the house soiling prob-lem. The lack of behaviors that indicate bonding (social play, allogrooming, sharing re-sources, and close proximity especially when the cats are relaxed) can also be indicative of problems between cats. This might prevent a cat from approaching and using a litter box if they feel threatened by another cat or simply feel uncomfort-able around its presence.[17,18]

Learned processes can greatly contribute to a cat not willingly using their litter box. Cats that experienced pain or fear while using it (such as cats with medical problems, anxiety disorders, those with social issues with other cats, or who have their litter boxes in a location of busy household traffic) or were uncomfortable about some fac-tor related to the management (such as a litter box that is poorly cleaned) might develop a learned aversion to their litter boxes. A secondary process that can develop is a learned preference for a new location, substrate, or both. As a cat tries to locate an alternative site to urinate, they might find another location or substrate more attractive (ie, cleaner, quieter, more private) and develop a strong preference that can significantly increase the complexity of the problem. A learned preference can remain even in the absence of the factor that led to the aversion in the first place.[22]

Urine Marking

Urine marking is a normal part of the feline social, agonistic, and communication repertoire. It is seen in cats that are sexually intact and neutered or spayed, in males and females, in confident and anxious cats.[9,14,15] In cats that are no longer intact (the majority of the US feline caseload), urine marking is largely caused by acute and chronic stress. Territorial and social issues are among the most common causes: cats that live in multicat households are at greater risk to present this behavior and often more than one cat does it.[23,24] The introduction of a new cat to a group can similarly cause cats to mark with urine. The same applies for household that have cats outside, regardless of the resident cats being strictly indoors or being allowed outdoors. Urine marking can also be seen in feline patients with anxiety conditions such as separation anxiety disorder, generalized anxiety disorder, and specific phobias. Schwartz[25] (2002) found that 75% of cats with separation anxiety marked their owner's bed with urine. One study showed that 52% of cats marking with urine had a recent change in their lives.[26] Urine marking episodes can coincide with FIC relapses because they are both triggered by stressors.[27] This is another example of a common type of multifactorial case where there are historical findings that evidence both urine marking and a medical condition that are concomitantly causing the cat to eliminate outside of the litter box.

TREATMENT

It should be clear at this point that not only multifactorial cases are frequent, but also that there is a common link among all problems that lead cats to miss their litter boxes: stress. Some of the treatment recommendations listed will address specific problems, but stress management and fulfilling cats' environmental needs are important on the management of all cases, including those caused by medical conditions.[28] Environmental enrichment has been shown to be one of the most effective tools to control clinical signs of FIC.[14,20] Treating any diagnosed medical conditions should be done immediately, or no recommended management changes and therapy will resolve the problem.

An initial problem that the practitioner might be faced with is the lack of evidence of which cat (or cats) are actually responsible for the urine spots found outside of the box. In multicat households, it is not rare for more than one cat to have a problem. A medical workup is required for all cats. Simple methods of identification include separating the cats in different areas of the house or monitoring them with a camera. The administration of oral or subcutaneous fluorescein dye has been recommended,[5,28] but its use is not always practical or possible and its results are not consistently reliable.

Litter Box Management

Much has been written about what is the ideal litter box management and the truth is that some cats are more flexible than others. This article reviews the recommendations found in the literature,[5,9,28] but individual differences and needs should be considered and discussed with clients. These recommendations apply for all feline patients, including those who present urine marking only.[29,30]

- Location and placement of boxes: Litter boxes should be placed in an area of the house that is, clean, quiet, and easily accessible to the cat. What that means can change during a cat's life. Having litter boxes in the basement might be fine for young and pain-free cats, but this might lead to problems when cats suffer from painful conditions (such as joint disease and FIC), difficult mobility (eg, obesity), cognitive and/or sensory decline, or medical problems that cause increased frequency and urgency to urinate (eg, FIC and other urinary tract problems). In these cases, cats should not need to use stairs to access their boxes and at least 1 box should be available close to the cat's preferred area in the house. The litter boxes should not be next to the cat's feeding station.

- If the household has more than 1 cat, often it is necessary that litter boxes are placed in more than 1 area to decrease the likelihood that a cat will miss the box owing to avoiding another cat.
- Dogs and children should not have access to the litter box area. Having a cat door installed or baby gate with a flap that only allows cats to pass can greatly help with management (**Fig. 1**). Appliances that produce sudden and/or loud noises should also be avoided next to litter boxes.
- Number of boxes: historically, the clinical behavioral medicine literature has recommended that clients should provide the same number of boxes as there are cats plus one additional box. As discussed before, this might not be necessary for every household but it is a sound rule. Some cats might use one box for defecation and one for urination.
- Size of boxes: 1.5 the length of the cat (from the nose to the base of the tail) has been recommended. This size should be enough to give a cat space to perform all active behaviors involved during toileting (digging, circling, squatting, and covering or burying). Often boxes available in pet shops are not large enough or have sides that are too high (which can be a problem for patients experiencing pain and discomfort). Large, rectangular storage boxes are ideal and affordable (**Fig. 2**). Boxes with shallower sides can help feline patients that have difficulty entering their current boxes. Cutting an entrance on taller boxes is an alternative solution.
- Type of boxes: Electronic or motion operated boxes are known for not providing appropriate hygiene and causing a stress or fear reaction in many cats. Covered boxes might trap smells, make some cats feel cornered or without an escape route, and might make clients less compliant when it comes to how often they scoop soiled litter. However, covered boxes can be useful for cats that mark inside of the box, urinate standing up, or are very enthusiastic diggers or buriers (**Fig. 3**). Large, rectangular storage boxes work well for most cats and are easy for clients to access and clean.

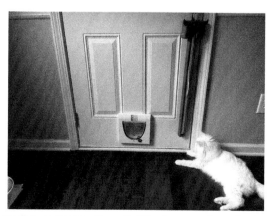

Fig. 1. Door with cat flap protecting the cat's litter box area from the household's traffic of people, children, and dogs.

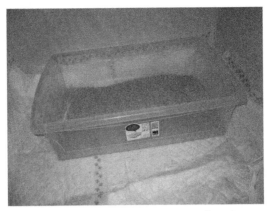

Fig. 2. Plastic storage box of appropriate size to serve as a litter box.

- Litter: Most cats do well with clay clumping litter. In the past, some studies suggested that nonscented litter was preferred by cats, but more recent publications showed no difference. That finding might have to do with the pet industry producing products with less aromatics, but considering the olfactory abilities of cat, it is sensible to advice clients to prefer litters that are less fragrant. Cats also differ in their preference for litter depth. At least 1.25 inches or 3 cm is recommended. Liners, slotted grills, and any deodorizing products should not be used, because cats have been shown to dislike them.
- Hygiene and cleaning management: Litter boxes should be scooped at least twice a day. The whole litter should be discarded and the box washed with soap and hot or warm water once a week. Strong chemicals and ammonia-based detergents or cleaners should not be used. Older plastic boxes (that might contain residual smell that is no longer removed after cleaning) need to be replaced by new boxes. No research has been done to evaluate how often in average this is necessary. The author recommends that a box is thrown away and replaced anytime that it seems to retain smell after being washed or is more than 2 years old.

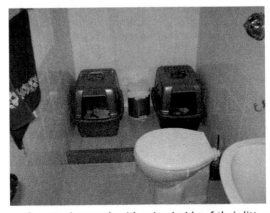

Fig. 3. Covered boxes for cats that mark with urine inside of their litter boxes.

- It might be helpful to trim perirectal and interdigital hair of long-haired cats. Please note that many cats will need to be desensitized and counterconditioned to the trimmer and the trimming procedure so that this is not a stressful process.

Addressing Social Problems Between Cats

If the elimination problem is being caused by conflict between cats (it does not matter if the problem in question is marking or toileting outside of the box), the client will need additional help. Many veterinarians are comfortable giving advice on intercat aggression, but others prefer to refer more complex cases to a veterinary behaviorist. As discussed, a comprehensive history is important so that all factors involved can be identified and treated. It is outside of the scope of this article to discuss intercat aggression, but separating the cats and providing individual resources[28,30] is good initial advice until the client can meet with a specialist.

Meeting a Cat's Environmental Needs

Environmental enrichment has been shown to be beneficial to brain health and welfare of several species (cats included) for decades.[31–34] From decreasing stress levels and clinical signs of anxiety in confinement situations to greatly contributing to treat medical problems where stress is an important factor (ie, FIC), there are several sources of scientific-based education for clients available to veterinarians.[9,35,36]

In 2013, the American Association of Feline Practitioners and the International Society of Feline Medicine published their feline environmental needs guidelines, which organized some of the main points (called the 5 pillars of a healthy feline environment) that should be addressed to provide cats with an environment that is as less stressful and more behaviorally fulfilling as possible.[37] These are as follows.

- Provide a safe place. Problem behaviors caused by fear and anxiety are often rooted in the cat's perception of having no control over their environment and relationships. Providing hiding areas and vertical or elevated areas also meets the cat biological need to observe their environment from above and help them find separation from cats that they do not get along with.
- Provide multiple and separated key environmental resources such as food, water, toileting, scratching, play, resting, and sleeping areas. Having separate resources and the ability to isolate themselves to perform important species-typical behaviors without feeling forced to interact with other cats can prevent conflict and stress-based behaviors.
- Provide opportunities for play and predatory behavior. It is long recognized by the literature that play behavior is important for mental health. Most cats also have a strong predatory drive. Being able to direct and fulfill these needs can prevent and control stress and anxiety (among other behavioral problems that are beyond the scope of this article). Functional toys that trigger both play and predatory behavior should always be available. Food toys are also highly recommended and beneficial for cats.
- Provide positive, consistent, and predictable human–cat social interaction. Predictability decreases fear and gives the cat a sense of control. Cats that are socialized to humans need their social and attachment needs fulfilled consistently.
- Provide an environment that respects the importance and sensitivity of the cat's sense of smell. When it comes to the problems addressed on this article, proper litter box management (especially in terms of hygiene and type of litter) is fundamental to avoid learned aversions to using their litter boxes.

Proper environmental enrichment benefits indoor cats' mental health and welfare; it also prevents and plays important role in the treatment of problem behaviors and medical conditions.[36] However, that cannot be compared with the complexity and stimulation of the outdoors environment. When the client has the means and the living situation allows for it, safe outdoors areas such catios and fenced enclosures should be considered (Dantas, personal observation; **Fig. 4**).

Stress Management and Removal of Triggers

For cats that mark with urine or toilet outside of their boxes owing to stressors in their environment, identifying and removing or managing these triggers is important for the resolution of the problem.[37] Depending on the problem at hand, this might include spaying and neutering intact animals, discouraging the presence of cats roaming outside, denying access to windows, keeping all cats indoors or separating resident cats temporarily (or permanently, see Having a difficult conversation). As explained, environmental enrichment greatly helps with stress management. Cats that suffer from anxiety disorders might need a referral to a veterinary behaviorist.

Behavior Therapy and Additional Management Changes

There is no place for punishment-based techniques when it comes to teaching a cat functional behaviors, especially when these arise from stress, fear, and anxiety.[28,30] The use of positive punishment such as spraying water or yelling (among others) should be discouraged in clients. These techniques will lead to fear and anxiety, and can trigger aggressive behavior toward other cats and people. Cats learn through operant conditioning the same way that dogs and other species do. When trying to get a cat to use their litter boxes again, providing positive reinforcement when the cat walks toward, sniffs around, jumps into, and/or uses the box can teach a positive association and reinforce the behavior without causing distress or harming the human–cat bond.[37]

Denying access to the areas marked or soiled can help with the process of getting the cat back to using the box (as long as all other techniques to address the primary problem and improve the cat's management are in place). That can be as simple as

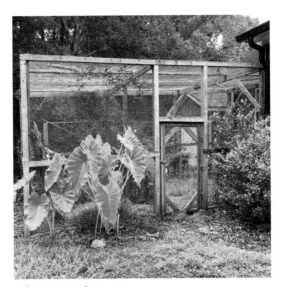

Fig. 4. Fenced in outdoor cat enclosure.

closing the door to the cat's current preferred location or removing a rug or mat from the floor. Aversive methods such as protecting furniture or other locations with materials that might discourage the cat (eg, aluminum foil paper, thick plastic, double-sided sticky tape, an upside down vinil runner) are acceptable as long as it does not make the cat more stressed and are done while the cause of the problem is being addressed (otherwise the cat will only change locations). Placing the cat's eating or drinking area on top of soiled areas or spraying areas with aversive smells and substances can be stressful and these methods are not necessarily effective. Soiled areas should be cleaned consistently with enzymatic cleaners. Placing a litter box on a preferred new area is not always practical or possible, but can help some cats go back to using their boxes.[9,28,30]

Pharmacologic Treatment of Stress, Fear, and Anxiety

As discussed, some cats that are marking or missing their litter boxes might have behavioral disorders or pathologies that involve fear and anxiety and therefore a dysfunctional neurochemistry. To this date, there is no US Food and Drug Administration–approved medication for the treatment of elimination problems in cats. However, many cats respond to treatment with serotoninergic drugs (eg, selective serotonin reuptake inhibitors, tricyclic antidepressants) and anxiolytics (eg, buspirone and benzodiazepines).[38–45] In 1 double-blind, placebo-controlled study, cats had a greater than 90% decrease in urine marking when receiving fluoxetine (administered orally at 1 mg/kg).[46]

Leslie Sinn's article, "Advances in Behavioral Psychopharmacology," in this issue, provides an updated review on treatment options for cats. Prescribing psychoactive medications involve owner education, caution with contraindications, side effects and drug interactions.

There is no need for treatment with psychoactive drugs when stress, fear and anxiety are not part of the problem (eg, toileting outside of the box owing to poor litter box hygiene). For other comprehensive reviews on psychopharmacology, drug use and dosing, consult Overall (2013)[47] and Crowell-Davis and Murray (2006).[48]

Encouraging Alternative Forms of Marking Behavior

Even though this method has not been evaluated scientifically, it is a common recommendation to encourage naturally occurring forms of marking that do not involve urine or feces (ie, bunting or facial rubbing and scratching). This might decrease the stress levels of cats that urine mark (and therefore decrease the frequency of urine marking episodes). Feliway has been used for this purpose[49] and toys especially designed to stimulate facial rubbing can be found on pet shops. Placing scratching posts in key areas is part of an optimum environmental needs management.[37]

How About Neutering or Spaying?

Neutering males can decrease urine marking by 78%.[50] However, neutered and spayed cats might urine mark which supports that sexual hormones and sexual behavior are not the only factors that regulate this behavior. In 1 study, 10% of males and 5% of females remained marking after sterilization.[51]

What Else Is Available?

The pet industry offers a plethora of options that promise to help with behavioral problems. From treats with calming herbs to homeopathy, essential oils, synthetic pheromones, wrapping clothing, and more, the truth is that there is insufficient scientific background and controlled studies for most products available.

Feliway (spray and diffuser) is claimed to be a "pheromone analogue" or a "synthetic version of the F3 fraction of the feline facial pheromone." Despite the controversy regarding its use owing to the limitations of most of studies published,[13,47,52] Feliway is frequently one of the first tools chosen by clients and feline practitioners, especially at the beginning of the problem.

A good number of prescription diets that have been formulated with ingredients that might help with anxiety and urinary tract problems are also available.[53,54] (see Jillian M. Orlando's article, "Behavioral Nutraceuticals and Diets," in this issue) for additional information.

Having a Difficult Conversation

Even though most cases of house soiling have good prognosis, in some circumstances despite the veterinarian's ability and the client's best efforts, the problem will not have full resolution without some tough decisions. For instance, cats that spray urine in response to stray or feral cats outside or to an internal conflict in the house might not stop even with pharmacologic treatment if the trigger is not completely removed from the environment. Clients might need to come with the terms of having to stop feeding or even deterring the presence of cats outside. Some cats can live a reasonably stress-free life while separated from each other in the house (and therefore might stop marking or toileting outside of their litter boxes), but unfortunately some will become even more distressed with the management changes. In these cases, rehoming the cat that for some reason triggers the house soiling problem on others is necessary.[55] It is part of the veterinarian's job to discuss realistic expectations and help clients to make the best possible decision with the cats' welfare in mind.

FOLLOW-UP

Once a treatment plan is designed for the patient, ideally the client should be contacted every 2 weeks until the problem is resolved.[9] This allows for the veterinarian to assess any problems or changes that need to be done to achieve the resolution of the problem.

PROGNOSIS

When the proper diagnosis is made (especially of behavioral origin without associated systemic diseases) and the appropriate treatment plan prescribed, the prognosis of feline elimination problems is good to excellent.

PREVENTION

Prevention and treatment go hand in hand when it comes to elimination problems in cats. Most of the techniques and measures recommended to treat feline patients are the same or similar to prevent that elimination problems happen in the first place. This is especially true for problems related to mental, emotional and behavioral health. Providing appropriate litter box management, addressing social issues between cats (by introducing them properly and managing problems early), eliminating sources of fear and anxiety in the cats' environment, and providing appropriate enrichment are all important to prevent that cats have reasons to quit using their litter boxes. This is lifesaving advice that should be part of the veterinarian's routine for cat appointments in general practice.[9]

REFERENCES

1. Patroneck GL, Glickman LT, Beck AM, et al. Risk factors for relinquishment of cats to an animal shelter. J Am Vet Med Assoc 1996;209(3):582–8.
2. Kogan L, New JG Jr, Kass PH, et al. Reasons for relinquishment of dogs and cats to 12 shelters. J Appl Anim Welf Sci 2000;3(2):93–106.
3. Scarlett JM, Salman MD, New JG Jr, et al. Behavioral reasons for relinquishment of companion animals in U.S. Animal Shelters: selected health and personal issues. J Appl Anim Welf Sci 1999;2(1):41–57.
4. Clifton M. Counts finds 5 million a year – AHA says 12 million. Animal People 1993;1:8.
5. Neilson J. Thinking outside the box: feline elimination. J Feline Med Surg 2004;6: 5–11.
6. Cooper LL. Feline inappropriate elimination. Vet Clin North Am Small Anim Pract 1997;27(3):569–600.
7. Houpt K. Housesoiling: treatment of a common feline problem. Vet Med 1991; 86(10):1000–6.
8. Seibert L. Animal behavior case of the month. J Am Vet Med Assoc 2004;224(10): 1594–6.
9. Carney HC, Sadek TP, Curtis TM, et al. AAFP and ISFM guidelines for diagnosing and solving house-soiling behavior in cats. J Feline Med Surg 2014;16:579–98.
10. Beaver BV. Feline eliminative behavior. In: Beaver BV, editor. Feline behavior: a guide for veterinarians. 2nd edition. St Louis (MO): Saunders; 2003. p. 247–73.
11. MacDonald DW, Apps PJ, Carr GM, et al. Social dynamics, nursing coalitions and infanticide among farm cats. Adv Ethol 1987;28:1–64.
12. Sarah LB, Bradshaw JWS. Communication in the domestic cat: within- and between-species. In: Turner DC, Bateson P, editors. The domestic cat. 3rd edition. New York: Cambridge University Press; 2014. p. 37–62.
13. Overall KL. Undesirable, problematic, and abnormal feline behavior and behavioral pathologies. In: Overall KL, editor. Manual of clinical behavioral medicine for dogs and cats. St Louis (MO): Elsevier; 2013. p. 360–456.
14. Scherk M. Urinary tract disorders. In: Little SE, editor. The cat clinical medicine and management. St Louis (MO): Elsevier; 2012. p. 935–1013.
15. Lascelles BD. Feline degenerative joint disease. Vet Surg 2010;39(1):2–13.
16. Sung W, Crowell-Davis SL. Elimination behavior patterns of domestic cats (*Felis catus*) with and without elimination behavior problems. Am J Vet Res 2006; 67(9):1500–4.
17. Bradshaw JWS, Casey RA, Brown SL. Communication. In: Bradshaw JWS, Casey RA, Brown SL, editors. The behaviour of the domestic cat. 2nd edition. Oxfordshire (United Kingdom): CABI; 2012. p. 91–112.
18. Bradshaw JWS, Casey RA, Brown SL. Undesired behaviour in the domestic cat. In: Bradshaw JWS, Casey RA, Brown SL, editors. The behaviour of the domestic cat. 2nd edition. Oxfordshire (United Kingdom): CABI; 2012. p. 190–205.
19. Buffington CA, Chew DJ, Kendall MS, et al. Clinical evaluation of cats with nonobstructive urinary tract diseases. J Am Vet Med Assoc 1997;210:46–50.
20. Buffington CAT, Westropp JL, Chew DJ. From FUS to Pandora syndrome. Where are we, how did we get here, and where to now? J Feline Med Surg 2014;16: 385–94.
21. Westropp JL, Kass PH, Buffington CA. Evaluation of the effects of stress in cats with idiopathic cystitis. Am J Vet Res 2006;67:731–6.
22. Overall KL. Diagnosing feline elimination disorders. Vet Med 1998;93(4):350–62.

23. Hart BL. Objectionable urine spraying and urine marking in cats: evaluation of progestin treatment in gonadectomized males and females. J Am Vet Med Assoc 1980;177(6):529–33.

24. Olm DD, Houpt KA. Feline house-soiling problems. Appl Anim Behav Sci 1988; 20(3–4):335–45.

25. Schwartz S. Separation anxiety syndrome in cats: 136 cases (1991-2000). J Am Vet Med Assoc 2002;220(7):1028–33.

26. Horwtiz DF. Behavioral and environmental factors associated with elimination behavior problems in cats: a retrospective study. Appl Anim Behav Sci 1997; 52(1–2):129–37.

27. Buffington CA. Comorbidity of interstitial cystitis with other unexplained conditions. J Urol 2004;170:1242–8.

28. Nielson JC. Feline house soiling: elimination and marking behaviors. Vet Clin North Am Small Anim Pract 2003;33(2):287–301.

29. Pryor PA, Hart BL, Bain MJ, et al. Causes of urine marking in cats and effects of environmental management on frequency of marking. J Am Vet Med Assoc 2001; 219(12):1709–13.

30. Horwitz DF, Neilson JC. House soiling: feline. In: Horwitz DF, Neilson JC, editors. Blackwell's five-minute veterinary consult clinical companion: canine & feline behavior. Ames (IA): Blackwell Publishing; 2007. p. 329–36.

31. Mellen J, MacPhee MS. Philosophy of environmental enrichment: past, present and future. Zoo Biol 2001;20:211–26.

32. Francis DD, Diorio J, Plotsky PM, et al. Environmental enrichment reverses the effects of maternal separation on stress reactivity. J Neurosci 2002;22(18):7840–3.

33. Rochlitz I. A review of the housing requirements of domestic cats (Felis silvestris catus) kept in the house. Appl Anim Behav Sci 2005;95:97–109.

34. Kry K, Casey R. The effect of hiding enrichment on stress levels and behavior of domestic cats (Felis sylvestris catus) in a shelter setting and the implications for adoption potential. Anim Welf 2007;16:375–83.

35. Ellis S. Environmental enrichment practical strategies for improving feline welfare. J Feline Med Surg 2009;11:901–12.

36. Dantas LMS, Delgado MM, Johnson I, et al. Food puzzles for cats: feeding for physical and emotional wellbeing. J Feline Med Surg 2016;18(9):723–32.

37. Ellis SL, Rodan I, Carney HC, et al. AAFP and ISFM feline environmental needs guidelines. J Feline Med Surg 2013;15:219–30.

38. Hart BL, Cliff KD, Tynes VV, et al. Control of urine marking by use of long-term treatment with fluoxetine or clomipramine in cats. J Am Vet Med Assoc 2005; 226(3):378–82.

39. Dehasse J. Feline urine spraying. Appl Anim Behav Sci 1997;52(3–4):365–71.

40. Hart BL, Eckstein RA, Powell KL, et al. Effectiveness of buspirone on urine spraying and inappropriate urination in cats. J Am Vet Med Assoc 1993;203(2):254–8.

41. Hart BL. Behavioral and pharmacologic approaches to problem urination in cats. Vet Clin North Am Small Anim Pract 1996;26(3):651–8.

42. Landsberg GM, Wilson AW. Effects of clomipramine in cats presented for urine marking. J Am Anim Hosp Assoc 2005;41:3–11.

43. King J, Steffan J, Heath S, et al. Determination of the dosage of clomipramine for the treatment of urine spraying in cats. J Am Vet Med Assoc 2004;225:881–7.

44. Romatowski J. Two cases of fluoxetine - responsive behavior disorders in cats. Feline Pract 1998;26(1):14–5.

45. Overall KL. Pharmacological treatment in behavioural medicine: the importance of neurochemistry, molecular biology and mechanistic hypotheses. Vet J 2001; 162(1):9–23.

46. Pryor PA, Hart BL, Cliff KD, et al. Effects of a selective serotonin reuptake inhibitor on urine spraying, behavior in cats. J Am Vet Med Assoc 2001;219(11):1557–61.

47. Overall KL. Pharmacological approaches to changing behavior and neurochemestry: roles for diet, supplements, nutraceuticals and medication. In: Overall KL, editor. Manual of clinical behavioral medicine for dogs and cats. St Louis (MO): Elsevier; 2013. p. 458–512.

48. Crowell-Davis SL, Murray T. Veterinary psychopharmacology. Ames (IA): Blackwell Publishing; 2006. p. 270.

49. Hunthausen W. Evaluating a feline facial pheromone analogue to control urine spraying. Vet Med 2000;95:151–5.

50. Hart BL, Barret RE. Effects of castration on fighting, roaming, and urine spraying in adult male cats. J Am Vet Med Assoc 1973;163(3):290–2.

51. Hart BL, Cooper L. Factors relating to urine spraying and fighting in prepubertally gonadectomized cats. J Am Vet Med Assoc 1984;184(10):1255–8.

52. Frank D, Beauchamp G, Palestrini C. Systematic review of the use of pheromones for treatment of undesirable behavior in cats and dogs. J Am Vet Med Assoc 2010;236(12):1308–16.

53. Scherk M. Concurrent disease management. In: Little SE, editor. The cat clinical medicine and management. St Louis (MO): Elsevier; 2012. p. 1098–133.

54. Landesberg G, Hunthausen W, Ackerman L. Feeding and diet-related problems. In: Landesberg G, Hunthausen W, Ackerman L, editors. 3rd edition. New York: Saunders; 2013. p. 151–61.

55. Landesberg G, Hunthausen W, Ackerman L. Feline housesoiling. In: Landesberg G, Hunthausen W, Ackerman L, editors. Behavior problems of the dog and cat. 3rd edition. New York: Saunders; 2013. p. 281–96.

Helping Pet Owners Change Pet Behaviors

An Overview of the Science

Beth Groetzinger Strickler, MS, DVM, CDBC

KEYWORDS

- Dominance • Learning • Punishment • Reinforcement • Trainer

KEY POINTS

- The relationship between pet and owner has changed significantly in recent years.
- The perception of pets as thinking, feeling beings has allowed a transition in training and care from one of poor and inadequate behavioral welfare to an approach that may allow seeing the full potential of patients.
- Veterinary professionals need to develop a solid understanding of evidence-based techniques for training and behavior modification.
- Veterinary professionals also need to begin to work with trainers and other behavior professionals who have the same mindset and goals and refer to a qualified professional if they do not have adequate knowledge.

DOMINANCE IN WOLVES AND DOGS: MYTH OR FACT?

For many years, the predominant approach to living with and training dogs (*Canis familiaris*) has been steeped in the theory of dominance and pack leadership. A dog who did not want to have his nails trimmed or a dog who would not come when called was labeled "dominant." This approach initially trickled out of the application of information gathered from the wolf (*Canis lupus*) community. Wolf packs were thought to maintain stability through an "alpha pair" (an alpha male and an alpha female), who were responsible for breeding and leadership of the group. Schenkel[1] initially suggested that the social relationship of the wolf was a yearly cyclic phenomenon. It was during this initial period that the pack became a closed society, the core of which involved the alpha pair. This theory maintained that other individuals in the pack would continuously vie for leadership but would be kept in their subordinate position by the higher-ranking individuals.[1,2] Schenkel developed his theory from observations of unrelated wolves in captivity at the Basel Zoological Garden, where up to 10 wolves were

Disclosure Statement: The author has nothing to disclose.
Veterinary Behavior Solutions, PO Box 4185, Johnson City, TN 37602, USA
E-mail address: beth.strickler.dvm@gmail.com

Vet Clin Small Anim 48 (2018) 419–431
https://doi.org/10.1016/j.cvsm.2017.12.008

maintained in a confined area. During his observation of this group, violent rivalries were observed. This information was then applied and compared with domestic dogs that were believed the most "primitive" (Eskimo dogs and street dogs). Schenkel's observation of these dog groups suggested that the group activity was not seasonal but instead remained static throughout the year.

For many years, the approach to group dynamics of both wolves and dogs was based on these assumptions. It was later determined that the artificial environment of a captive group of wolves was not representative of the natural assemblage of wolves. A family of wolves is composed of a breeding pair and their juvenile offspring from the previous 1 year to 3 years, and a group of wolves may sometimes include more than 1 family. As the young wolves mature, they typically begin to disperse between the ages of 1 and 2, with few remaining past the age of 3 years.[3] The contrast of this fluid family unit to the artificial captive pack that is required to live in close proximity for many years was stark. An analogy has been made by Mech[3,4] that comparing wolves in captivity with natural packs is equivalent to studying human family dynamics with information from humans in refugee camps.

Unfortunately, this distorted information was applied to the management of domestic dogs as well as some other species. This perspective was used to view both the relationship between pets and owners and between pets living in the same home. In the popular press, professional approach, and in the home, the usage of dominance theory became an ingrained and acceptable approach for all behavioral issues. The approach to treat a canine behavioral problem became "be a pack leader" or the "alpha" in the home.

More recently, observation of natural wolf packs has demonstrated that the group is not a rigid, force-based dominance hierarchy as originally believed. Posturing is evident between dogs during social interactions, consistent with dominant and submissive gestures. But it is generally thought that both active and passive submissive interactions help promote friendly interactions and decrease conflict.[1,3,5] Additionally, the exchanges of agonistic and submissive signaling have not been correlated with dominance, even in wolves.[6] The current view more closely adheres to the theory that the wolf pack is a family unit with the adult breeding parents guiding the group activities; yet each wolf is an individual with flexibility consistent with that found in humans.

The remaining question is whether information from natural and/or captive wolf packs can be applied to the domesticated dog. Evidence that domesticated dogs are significantly different from wolves, in their domestication as well as in social cognition, has further removed probable comparisons between wolves and dogs.[7–9] Although multiple examples of how dogs differ from wolves exist, a common life example of the significant differences between wolves and dogs can be demonstrated by evaluation of barking behaviors. Although both dogs and wolves bark, the threshold for barking is lower in dogs, the patterns have more variability in dogs, and dogs bark in various social situations. Studies have indicated that humans' selection over time has altered some traits of individual dogs. Often selection for a particular trait has been strengthened in a breed over time, sometimes increasing or decreasing a behavior that is less compatible with the home environment.

Historical use of the term, *dominant*, in describing an individual animal has led pet owners and trainers alike to react and interact with their pets in a particular way. The thought that dominance is a personality trait of individuals dogs, and that a dog's goal is to achieve resource control, has allowed humans to react in such a way to adjust the relationship through physical coerciveness. Research has shown that there is no evidence that dominance is character trait of individual dogs. Instead, dominance can be defined as a property of a relationship that results from asymmetry in personality traits between dogs.[10–12]

The concept that a dog's interaction with humans and other dogs is based on a motivation to achieve status cannot be supported through current evidence. Dogs do not compete for right of access to resources, regardless of their current or future value. This is based in part on the supposition that dogs have not been shown to be aware of the relational discrepancy between themselves and other dogs (ie, their own status). Additionally, companion dogs in homes do not have to compete to stay alive as those they have been compared with (free-ranging dogs, feral dogs, and wolves). The relationships that dogs have with people in the home are a product of their successive interactions over time in addition to their genetic predisposition. A model of developmental social competence[13] identifies a dog's ability to interact in dyadic relationships in its world. The relationship between humans and dogs is now considered similar in some functional ways to the infant-parent attachment that occurs in humans (**Box 1**).

PROVIDING A PREDICTABLE ENVIRONMENT FOR LEARNING

Science has allowed glimpses that companion animals are more complicated than a simple hierarchical approach allows. Although multiple major organizations have published position statements contrary to the dominance theory,[14,15] the techniques have persisted in the general public. To understand how to be more successful in living with pets, communicating well with a pet and influencing the pet's behavior when needed, it is important to start with an understanding of how pets learn. A study of how human individuals learn has been pursued for centuries, tracing back as early as the French

---

Box 1
Quick view terminology

Learning: a process whereby an organism is changed

Positive reinforcement: adding something the animal likes to increase the likelihood that the behavior will recur

Negative reinforcement: removal of something unpleasant, which increases the likelihood that the behavior will recur

Positive punishment: presentation of something undesirable, which decreases the behavior

Negative punishment: involves the removal of something desirable, which causes the behavior to decrease

DRA: differential reinforcement of alternative behavior

DRI: differential reinforcement of incompatible behavior

Aversive techniques: techniques that cause pain, fear, or anxiety, such as pinch/prong collars, choke collars, electronic/shock collars, alpha rolls, and dominance downs

Nonaversive techniques: techniques that identify and reward desirable behaviors using rewards, play, and nonconfrontational interactions

Continuous reinforcement: a behavior is rewarded each time it occurs; best used when teaching a new behavior

Intermittent reinforcement: a behavior is rewarded in intermittent ratios or intervals; best used to maintain a behavior

philosopher René Descartes in the 1600s.[16] Research has been answering this question for many years in the field of psychology.

Living with a dog involves a degree of interaction that is beyond obedience training. Previously it has been recommended that interactions with dogs follow a predictable leadership structure that involves regimented interactions requiring the dog to "defer" to the owner to receive all resources it considers valuable (referred to as Nothing in Life is Free or No Free Lunch Principle).[17] Although these approaches to interaction with canine companions have improved many behaviors and been a significant part of behavior modification, limiting interactions with pets to a simplistic structure such as this may be naïve and simplistic. It has been proposed that Nothing in Life is Free–type programs have caused poor welfare when followed to the extreme, resulting in restriction of required resources in the environment. The application of this technique is best used in combination with an understanding of the relationship that occurs when dogs and humans live in community.

EARLY TRAINING TECHNIQUES

Early records of training based on dominance beliefs can be traced to the work of Colonel Konrad Most during the early 1900s.[18] Most's training manual encouraged techniques that resulted in complete surrender of the dog to the human. Statements, such as, "The switch should be employed until the animal submits and his will to resist, and the exasperation that accompanies it, is replaced by fear,"[(p36)] created a culture of training that has been hard to redirect. These techniques permeated through the public and scientific literature for years and still exist in some popular media. Techniques that involve confrontation, domination, and punishment have included such techniques as hitting and kicking dogs, growling at a dog, physically forcing the release of an item from a dog, staring at a dog, using an alpha roll (forcibly turning a dog onto the back until it submits), grabbing by scruff or jowls, throwing items at dogs, and/or corrections with collars or electronic devices. Usage of antiquated dominance-based approaches has led clients to use techniques that are seen as confusing, intimidating, threatening, and/or confrontational.[19] The transition over recent years to a perception of a dog as a companion (as opposed to property) has allowed for dominance-based approaches to be slowly replaced by evidence-based practices.

An owner's perception of the role of a dog in the home influences the methods and approach used when training the dog. If a dog is perceived as a creature attempting to move up a hierarchy and gather and defend resources, the approach taken when addressing a behavior problem is to attempt to create submission or change the rank of the dog. If the dog is instead viewed as a companion with intelligence and emotions, the approach to addressing unwanted behaviors is quite different. Pregowski[20] has suggested that adhering to a strict limit of behaviorism will decrease the relationship that can and does occur with pets. If the relationship is instead viewed as a "bilateral bond of mutual benefit," with the humans as guides and partners in the training, a different path will be taken.

Evidence-based training has its roots in the field of psychology, where learning has been systematically evaluated in the laboratory for years. Learning has been demonstrated to occur in multiple ways: as a result of association with experiences or events, through consequences that follow the action, and through observation and cooperative learning. Years of research have provided a knowledge base of learning theory from which to base the training of canine companions and working dogs. It allows understanding how learning occurs. Creation of a behavior modification plan for a patient begins with identification of the learning that has previously occurred and design of a new learning (treatment) plan based on scientific principles. Unfortunately, the decision to use a particular technique has not historically been dependent only on evidence of effectiveness available.[21] Individuals in the training and veterinary community have relied on general experience, recommendations from individuals in the training community, or commonality (how often technique is used in region). To make the shift to evidence-based techniques, a solid understanding of learning theory is imperative.

HOW DO DOGS LEARN BEST?

Although many veterinary staff avoid discussing behavioral issues with clients because they are unfamiliar with the terminology of learning theory, a basic understanding of learning theory is necessary for working effectively with animals with and without behavioral issues. Every interaction with an animal results in learning. It is important that veterinary professionals understand the science behind how animals learn (both deliberately and accidentally) and that veterinary professionals understand how to teach patients new information.

Learning is a process whereby an organism is changed. In animals, learning is typically monitored by external behaviors, although there is an internal process that occurs as well. The process of learning depends on an animal's perception, an animal's memory, and an animal's ability to categorize events as similar or dissimilar to previous events. An animal's behavioral response (or evidence of learning) depends on the animal's physical ability to perform the response, the animal's motivation to respond to the learning session, the animal's emotional arousal level at the time of request for response, the animal's opportunity for response, and whether learning truly has occurred. It has been noted by previous investigators that when individuals enroll in an obedience class or training program for a pet, they do not anticipate that they (the humans) will be the ones receiving education.[22] But educating an owner to understand and recognize when and how learning occurs allows for a more fluent process of behavior change and cooperation.

LEARNING TERMINOLOGY AND TECHNIQUES

A solid foundation in learning theory starts with an understanding of the 2 common types of learning. *Classical conditioning* is the repeated pairing of a neutral stimulus (that has no preexisting meaning for the animal) with another stimulus that causes a reflexic response, which results in a learned (conditioned) response. The well-known laboratory example of classical conditioning occurred when Ivan Pavlov was studying the salivary reflex in dogs. He noticed the dogs began salivating when the assistant walked into the room because they had learned to associate the assistant with the presentation of food.[23] A common conditioned response in people is the pairing of an emotional response (being in love) with a particular song. Many individuals have experienced a particular song playing on the radio and an emotional memory instantly activated.

Operant conditioning involves learning that a consequence (positive or negative) occurs with an action. In this situation, the animal causes the results; what the animal does is critical to what happens next. The likelihood of a behavior increases if it is reinforced or decreases if it is punished. Reinforcement and punishment are entirely in the eye of the animal.

Companion animals are learning all the time—intentionally or unintentionally. In the real world of animal behavior, classical and operant learning can occur simultaneously. For example, even though a dog associates the sound of the can opener with food and begins to salivate at the sound of it (classical conditioning), it is then rewarded for coming to the food bowl with the food (operant conditioning).

Operant conditioning can be broken down into 4 subtypes of learning.[16,24] *Positive reinforcement* involves adding something the animal likes to increase the likelihood that the behavior will recur. For example, an owner says "sit," the dog sits and the dog is given a treat. The treat serves to increase the likelihood of the response in the future. A reinforcer is a "reward." Reward implies that it is good and that both the giver and the receiver consider it a reward. If this is true, reinforcing a behavior increases the likelihood of its occurrence.

Many in the research community have considered what is "rewarding" for dogs. In a comparison of shelter dogs, owned dogs, and hand-reared wolves, brief social interaction was found ineffective reinforcement when compared with food.[25] An extended history of reinforcement with the owner did not affect the reinforcing effect of the social interaction. A comparison of food reward, petting a dog, and vocal praise indicated that the food reward shortened the time taking for the command to be completed during the early stages of training.[26] Alternatively, a preference for vocal praise versus food was found when evaluating dogs who had been trained to enter a functional MRI awake.[27] In all the studies, individual differences were found. Because food delivery in training almost always involves social interaction, it is hard to separate and differentiate the effect of each. In the previous study, some dogs did find food more rewarding and some did find social interaction more rewarding, but social reinforcement is important. Other studies have shown that dogs prefer petting to vocal praise in both shelter and owned dogs.[28] There was additionally no satiation effect with petting that sometimes is seen with food delivery. In each situation with an individual patient, it is important to evaluate the appropriate motivator for that patient.[29] Additionally, the reward system may need to be adjusted over time due to satiation or changes in stage of learning or interaction and increased when faced with very arousing stimuli.

Evaluation of a dog's ability to learn based on these theories of learning have indicated that identification of what is rewarding may be different dependent on the task being learned and the individual dog. Obedience for the commands to "give" or "leave" an object was found significantly greater if a dog was trained with play as reward (vs any other method). Obedience for "heel" was also significantly greater for dogs using praise as reward.[30] Identification of the function of a behavior (known as functional analysis) prevents a clinician from assigning a standard treatment that may not address a dog's problem behavior. Instead, identifying the function of the behavior allows the clinician to target the reward system that is maintaining the behavior. For example, a dog who is barking may be rewarded by the attention an owner gives when yelling at the dog to stop barking.[31]

Many trainers and behaviorists use clicker training as a tool in behavior modification under the supposition that clicker training facilitates task acquisition more quickly.[32,33] Clicker training uses a handheld signaling device (a clicker), which emits an audible noise when pressed. The click is emitted when the animal performs a desired behavior and is typically followed by a food reward.[34] The clicker has been proposed to be a secondary reinforcer by pairing the clicker with the primary reinforcer (typically food). Chiandetti and colleagues[35] found no differences in acquisition found between a verbal marker (eg, "bravo"), food dispensing alone, and use of a clicker. The study used experienced trainers, who were instructed to give a social cue of a bow prior to dispension of the food only. It is possible that the social cue served as a secondary reinforcer or cue for the dispension of the food, creating a similar scenario to the clicker scenario. For many trainers, professional and nonprofessional, clicker training may serve as a valuable tool in the acquisition of the behavior.

Positive reinforcement is the most common type of operant conditioning used in most training today.[36] Other techniques may be incorporated effectively into a behavior modification program when used appropriately. *Negative reinforcement*, another subcategory of operant conditioning, involves the removal of something unpleasant when a behavior is performed that increases the likelihood that the behavior will recur. For example, a dog is asked to "sit" while pushing on his rump, the dog sits, and the hand is removed from the rump. This also increases the likelihood of the behavior occurring in the future.

Punishment results in a behavior occurrence decreasing with the presentation or removal of something undesirable. *Positive punishment* involves the presentation of something undesirable when a behavior is performed. Because the consequence is undesirable, the behavior decreases. Positive punishment must occur within seconds of the behavior to be effective. Unfortunately, the average pet owner is typically not able to be consistent in response to a pet and is often unable to determine an appropriate intensity of consequence that fits within the scientific definition of punishment.[16] This may result in punishment applied with poor accuracy and/or ineffectively by the individual delivering the punishment and can cause an increase in anxiety, fear, and aggression. Incorrect usage of positive punishment may be a result of poor timing of the punishment. Additionally, in some circumstances, anxiety or fear may be associated with the individual delivering the punishment. Logistically, positive punishment does not provide an alternative behavior for the animal. An example of a commonly used technique that may be classified as positive punishment results when an owner attempts to decrease the behavior of a dog jumping on visitors by delivering a knee to the chest (note: this is not recommended because many dogs who are punished learn to fear the punisher or shut down in training [discussed previously]). *Negative punishment* involves the removal of something considered desirable by the pet as a consequence for the behavior, which causes the behavior to decrease. For example, a puppy is playing too roughly and the owner stands up, leaves the area, and stops play; the puppy's rough playing therefore decreases.

An alternative approach to focusing on the undesired behaviors is to instead reinforce a more appropriate alternative behavior. Differential reinforcement of alternative behavior and differential reinforcement of incompatible behavior are effective ways to reduce a problem behavior.[37] Obedience for not chewing objects was greater for those that received alternative objects to chew versus any other method.[30] Persistence on an unsolvable task allows for observation of alternative behaviors that occur when a previously reinforced response is placed on extinction.[31]

AVOIDING THE PUNISHMENT TRAP

As changes in training techniques have occurred, evaluations of efficacy and discussion of welfare have permeated both the animal and human literature. Two recent large literature reviews of studies evaluating efficacy and effects of aversive-based training methods suggest that aversive-based training can negatively influence dog welfare and dog-human interactions.[38,39] Several of the reviewed studies have shown that the aversive techniques may result in increased symptoms of stress and/or decreased interactions with people. Fernandes and colleagues[38] noted that conclusions were limited by the fact that many of the studies were survey-based studies with owner reports rather than objective data. Empirical studies were mainly evaluations of electronic collar training. Ziv[39] evaluated a slightly different literature review related to 17 previous studies involving punishment and punishment type techniques. Although Ziv limited the review to only those studies that compared 2 or more training methods, there was significant overlap with the Fernandes and colleagues review, with 12 of the studies appearing in both reviews. Ziv found that aversive training methods often have undesirable and unintended outcomes, which puts dogs' welfare at risk. There was no evidence that aversive training methods were more effective.

A positive correlation between punishment and problematic behaviors has been identified both in animals and humans.[30,40] A survey of dog owners making an appointment at a behavioral referral center indicated a positive relationship between utilization of confrontational methods (such as hitting, kicking, alpha roll, and physical reprimands) and an aggressive response from the dog.[41] Dogs who had received shocks from an electronic training collar in the past showed more stress-related behaviors than control (nonshocked) dogs in a study of German Shepherd dogs.[42] Dogs whose owners reported to use a higher level of punishment were less likely to interact with strangers and tended to be less playful.[43] Deldalle and Gaunet[44] evaluated walking on a leash and obeying a "sit" command with well-trained owned dogs using either a negative reinforcement–based method (such as removal of an aversive leash correction/pressure) or a positive reinforcement–based method (such as a food reward). Dogs in this study showed increased signs of stress (mouth licking, yawning, scratching, sniffing, shivering, and whining) and lowered body postures with the negative reinforcement–based methods whereas dogs showed increased attentiveness toward the owner with positive reinforcement–based methods. Dogs whose owners tended to use more rewards in training tended to perform better in a novel training task.[43] Dogs whose owners used punishment-based collars reported less satisfaction with their dogs' behaviors.[45] Therefore, when creating a treatment plan or training a pet, the least invasive/minimally aversive (LIMA) approach is likely the best choice.

WHAT ELSE IS KNOWN ABOUT HOW DOGS LEARN?

Although much of the literature on learning in companion animals has previously focused on theories of classical and operant conditioning, more recently a cognitive approach has begun to permeate the literature in an attempt to define what occurs during the canine mental process and the human-dog interaction. There is evidence that multiple factors of the human-dog interaction affect a dog's ability to process and learn,[46] including but not limited to the body position of the human,[47] eye contact or attention,[48,49] and proximity.[50] So instead of evaluating a dog's behavior and modifying it through a direct associative approach (event 1 activates or predicts event 2), a more current approach allows a clinician or trainer to include processing biases and variations in attention dependent on the situation or patient.

Another variant of social learning has been evaluated by studying the efficacy of a "do as I do" (DAID) method. DAID involves a demonstration by the owner of the action the dog is requested to perform followed by a command to "do it." This process is repeated until success is achieved. The DAID method was compared with shaping, with use of clicker training in performance of simple and complex tasks.[51] The DAID and shaping/clicker training techniques were comparable for simple tasks, but DAID improved performance in complex actions or series of actions. Fugazza and Miklosi[52] also found that the DAID strategy improved performance in object-related tasks (such as opening a sliding door) and may have been mildly beneficial with body movement tasks (such as jumping in the air). DAID also seems to enhance the process of generalization and it has been thought that it may equate to a 12-month-old infant's mental representations of others' actions.

HOW AND WHEN TO INVOLVE A TRAINER

An individual's lack of knowledge, difficulty in following a behavior modification plan, and continuity between individuals interacting with a pet may create a barrier to implementation of a behavior treatment plan. Because timing has been shown important in learning of behaviors,[53] and consistency in owner behavior is related to better obedience,[54] consistency and accuracy of training may be important skills that can be difficult for inexperienced owners or those with physical disabilities to accomplish well. Owners who engaged in informal training at home and did not attend formal training were more likely to report some form of aggression in their dogs.[55] Generalization is often an overlooked part of training by nonprofessionals.[56] Additionally, maintaining an adequate level of motivation to engage in training with a typical client's busy lifestyle may be difficult. Therefore, involving a skilled trainer in the behavior treatment plan may accelerate and potentially improve the results for behavior modification.[57]

An excellent and skilled trainer may be able to help a client identify appropriate motivators, help set up scenarios where both dog and client can be successful, and set realistic expectations. The trainer may also be able to help the client determine if a dog understands what a client is asking of the dog and can help adjust a plan that may be creating frustration for either client or patient (**Boxes 2** and **3**).

Box 2
How to select a dog trainer

Is the trainer using scientifically based training (potential key words to look for: reward-based training, force-free, and humane-training methods)?

Is the trainer a good teacher? Can the trainer communicate well with both humans and pets?

Is the trainer participating in continuing education?

Is the trainer requiring a relationship with a veterinarian (either for routine medical care, such as vaccines, and/or a medical evaluation for behavior problem)?

Is the trainer a member of or certified by a professional organization (**Box 3** lists some possibilities)? (Note: certification does not ensure technique.)

Does the trainer have insurance?

Visit a class (evaluate cleanliness and trainer's interaction with clients and pets).

Walk away if
    Trainer uses choke collar, pinch collar, or electronic/shock collar.
    Trainer bans head collars of any kind.
    Trainer recommends physical reprimands of any kind (hitting, kicking, pinching, and so forth).
    Trainer uses word "alpha" or "dominant."

Box 3
What do all those letters mean?

- DACVB—Diplomate of the American College of Veterinary Behaviorists
- CTC—Certificate in Training and Counseling from Academy for Dog Trainers
- KPA CTP—Karen Pryor Academy Certified Training Partner
- CPDT-KA, CPDT-KSA, CBCC-KA—assessed by the Certification for Professional Dog Trainers
- IAABC—International Association of Animal Behavior Consultants
  - CDBC—Certified Dog Behavior Consultant
  - CCBC—Certified Cat Behavior Consultant
  - CHBC—Certified Horse Behavior Consultant
  - CPBC—Certified Parrot Behavior Consultant
- CAAB—Certified Applied Animal Behaviorists (certified by Animal Behavior Society)
- CTT-A, PCT-A, or PCBC-A—assessed by the Pet Professional Accreditation Board (operated by Pet Professional Guild)
- APDT—Association of Professional Dog Trainers—membership—uses LIMA

Abbreviations: CBCC, Certified Behavior Consultant Canine; CTT-A, Canine Training Technician (Accredited); KA, knowledge assessed; KSA, knowledge and skills assessed; LIMA, least intrusive, minimally aversive; PCBC-A, Professional Canine Behavior Consultation (Accredited); PCT-A, Professional Canine Trainer (Accredited)

SUMMARY

The relationship between pet and owner has changed significantly in recent years. The perception of companion animals as thinking, feeling beings has allowed a transition in training and care from one of poor and inadequate behavioral welfare to an approach that may allow seeing the full potential of patients.[58] Veterinary professionals need to develop a solid understanding of evidence-based techniques for training and behavior modification, need to begin to work with trainers and other behavior professionals who have the same mindset and goals, and refer to a qualified professional if they do not have adequate knowledge. Veterinarians take an oath to use "scientific knowledge and skills for the benefit of society through the protection of animal health and welfare" (American Veterinary Medical Association).[59] Empirical data are available for a movement from dominance-based interactions to evidence-based practices in veterinary behavior that improve the health and welfare of these patients.

REFERENCES

1. Schenkel R. Expression studies on wolves: captivity observations. Behavior 1947; 1:81–129.
2. Rabb GB, Woolpy JH, Ginsburg BE. Social relationships in a group of captive wolves. American Zoologist 1967;7:305–11.
3. Mech LD. Alpha status, dominance and division of labor in wolf packs. Can J Zool 1999;77:1196–203. Jamestown (ND): Northern Prarie Wildlife Research Center Home Page. (version 16MAY2000). Available at: http://www.npwrc.usgs.Gov/resource/2000/alstat/alstat.htm.
4. Mech LD. Leadership in wolf, canis lupus, packs. Can Field Nat 2000;114(2):250–63.
5. Bernstein IS. Dominance: the baby and the bathwater. Behav Brain Sci 1981;4:419–57.
6. Lockwood R. Dominance in wolves: useful contruct or bad habit?. In: Klinghammer E, editor. The behavior and ecology of wolves. New York: Garland STPM Press; 1979. p. 225–44.

7. Bradshaw JWS, Blackwell EJ, Casey RA. Dominance in domestic dogs-useful construct or bad habit? J Vet Behav 2009;4:135–44.

8. Overall KL. Manual of clinical behavioral medicine for dogs and cats. St Louis (MO): Mosby; 2013. p. 122–61.

9. Miklosi A. Affiliative and agonistic social relationships. In: Dog behaviour, evolution and cognition. 2nd edition. Oxford: Oxford University Press; 2015. p. 223–51.

10. Pachel C. Leadership dos and don'ts for dogs. AAHA Long Beach 2010 Proceedings. Scientific, Management and Technician Programs. Long Beach (CA), March 18–21, 2010.

11. Reisner I. Moving beyond "Leader of the Pack": changing dog behavior using science instead of myth. Today's Veterinary Practice 2014;46–9.

12. Bradshaw JWS, Blackwell EJ, Casey RA. Dominance in domestic dogs – a response to Schilder et al (2014). J Vet Behav 2016;11:102–8.

13. Miklósi A, Topál J. What does it take to become 'best friends'? Evolutionary changes in canine social competence. Trends Cogn Sci 2013;17(6):287–94.

14. American Veterinary Society of Animal Behavior. In: AVSAB Position statement on the use of dominance theory in behavior modification of animals. Available at: https://avsab.org/resources/position-statements/. Accessed October 8, 2017.

15. The Association of Professional Dog Trainers. In: Dominance and dog training. Available at: https://apdt.com/about/position-statements/. Accessed October 8, 2017.

16. Schwartz B, Robbins SJ. Psychology of learning and behavior. 4th edition. New York: WW Norton & Company; 1995. p. 21–9, 171–205.

17. Voith VL, Borchelt PL. Diagnosis and treatment of dominance aggression in dogs. Vet Clin North Am Small Anim Pract 1982;12(4):655.

18. Most CK. Training dogs: a manual. London: Popular Dogs Publishing; 1954. p. 36.

19. Browne CM, Starkey NJ, Foster TM, et al. Examination of the accuracy and applicability of information in popular books on dog training. Soc Anim 2017;25:411–35.

20. Pregowski MP. Your dog is your teacher: contemporary dog training beyond radical behaviorism. Soc Anim 2015;23:525–43.

21. Friedman SG. What's wrong with this picture? Effectiveness is not enough. Journal of Applied Companion Animal Behavior 2009;3(1):41–5.

22. Greenebaum JB. Training dogs and training humans: symbolic interaction and dog training. Anthrozoos 2010;23(2):129–41.

23. Reid PJ. Excel-erated Learning: explaining in plain English how dogs learn and how best to teach them. Berkeley (CA): James & Kenneth Publishers; 1996.

24. Mills DS. Learning, training and behaviour modification techniques. In: Horwitz DF, Mills DS, Heath S, editors. BSAVA manual of canine and feline behaviour medicine. Gloucester (UK): British Small Animal Veterinary Association; 2002. p. 37–48.

25. Feuerbacher EN, Wynne CDL. Relative efficacy of human social interaction and food as reinforcers for domestic dogs and hand-reared wolves. J Exp Anal Behav 2012;98(1):105–29.

26. Fukuzawa M, Hayashi N. Comparison of 3 different reinforcements of learning in dogs (Canis familiaris). J Vet Behav 2013;8:221–4.

27. Cook PF, Prichard A, Spivak M, et al. Awake canine fMRI predicts dogs' preference for praise vs food. Soc Cogn Affect Neurosci 2016;11(12):1853–62.

28. Feuerbacher EN, Wynne CDL. Shut up and pet me! Domestic dogs (Canis lupus familiaris) prefer petting to vocal praise in concurrent and single-alternative choice procedures. Behav Process 2015;110:47–59.

29. Feuerbacher EN, Wynne CDL. Most domestic dogs (Canis lupus familiaris) prefer food to petting: Population, context and schedule effect in concurrent choice. J Exp Anal Behav 2014;101(3):385–405.

30. Hiby EF, Rooney NJ, Bradshaw JWS. Dog training methods: their use, effectiveness and interaction with behaviour and welfare. Anim Welf 2004;13:63–9.

31. Hall NJ. Persistence and resistance to extinction in the domestic dog: Basic research and applications to canine training. Behav Process 2017;141:67–74.

32. Pryor K. Don't shoot the dog! The new art of teaching and training. 2nd edition. New York: Bantam Books; 1999.

33. Pfaller-Sadovsky N, Medina LG, Hurtado-Parrado C. It's mine! Using clicker training as a treatment of object guarding in four companion dogs (Canis lupus familiaris). J Vet Behav 2017. https://doi.org/10.1016/j.jveb.2017.08.002.

34. Feng LC, Howell TJ, Bennett PC. How clicker training works: comparing reinforcing, marking, and bridging hypotheses. Appl Anim Behav Sci 2016;181:34–40.

35. Chiandetti C, Avella S, Fongaro E, et al. Can clicker training facilitate conditioning in dogs? Appl Anim Behav Sci 2016;184:109–16.

36. Alexander MB, Friend T, Haug L. Obedience training effects on search dog performance. Appl Anim Behav Sci 2011;132:152–9.

37. Cooper JO, Heron TE, Heward WL. Applied behavior analysis. 2nd edition. Upper Saddle River (NJ): Pearson; 2007. p. 469–84.

38. Fernandes JG, Olsson IAS, deCastro ACV. Do aversive-based training methods actually compromise dog welfare?: a literature review. Appl Anim Behav Sci 2017. https://doi.org/10.1016/j.applanim.2017.07.001.

39. Ziv G. The effectsof using aversive training methods in dogs – a review. J Vet Behav 2017;19:50–60.

40. MacKenzie MJ, Nicklas E, Waldfogel J, et al. Spanking and child development across the first decade of life. Pediatrics 2013;132(5):e1118–25.

41. Herron ME, Shofer FS, Reisner IR. Survey of the use and outcome of confrontational and non-confrontational training methods in client-owned dogs showing undesired behaviors. Appl Anim Behav Sci 2009;117:47–54.

42. Schilder MBH, van der Borg JAM. Training dogs with help of the shock collar: short and long term behavioural effects. Appl Anim Behav Sci 2004;35:319–34.

43. Rooney NJ, Cowan S. Training methods and owner-dog interactions: Links with dog behaviour and learning ability. Appl Anim Behav Sci 2011;132:169–77.

44. Deldalle S, Gaunet F. Effects of 2 training methods on stress-related behaviors of the dog (Canis familiaris) and on the dog-owner relationship. J Vet Behav 2014;9: 58–65.

45. Kwan JT, Bein MJ. Owner attachment and problem behaviors related to relinquishment and training techniques of dogs. J Appl Anim Welf Sci 2013;16: 168–83.

46. Haselgrove M. Overcoming associative leaerning. J Comp Psychol 2016;130(3): 226–40.

47. Fukuzawa M, Mills DS, Cooper JJ. More than just a word: non-semantic command variables affect obedience in the domestic dog (Canis familiaris). Appl Anim Behav Sci 2005;91:129–41.

48. Schwab C, Huber L. Obey or not obey? Dogs (Canis familiaris) behave differently in response to attentional states of their owners. J Comp Psychol 2006;120(3): 169–75.

49. Virányi Z, Topál J, Gácsi M, et al. Dogs respond appropriately to cues of humans' attentional focus. Behav Process 2004;66(2):161–72.
50. Gerencser L, Kosztolanyi A, Delanoeije J, et al. The effect of reward-handler dissociation on dogs' obedience performance in different conditions. Appl Anim Behav Sci 2016;174:103–10.
51. Fugazza C, Miklosi A. Should old dog trainers learn new tricks? The efficiency of the Do as I do method and shaping/clicker training method to train dogs. Appl Anim Behav Sci 2014;153:53–61.
52. Fugazza C, Miklosi A. Social learning in dog training: The effectiveness of the do as I do method compared to shaping/clicker training. Appl Anim Behav Sci 2015; 171:146–51.
53. Payne EM, Bennett PC, McGreevy PD. DogTube: an examination of dogmanship online. J Vet Behav 2017;17:50–61.
54. Arhant C, Bubna-Littitz H, Bartels A, et al. Behaviour of smaller and larger dogs: Effects of training methods, inconsistency of owner behaviour and level of engagement in activities with the dog. Appl Anim Behav Sci 2010;123:131–42.
55. Blackwell EJ, Twells C, Seawright A, et al. The relationship between training methods and the occurrence of behavior problems, as reported by owners, in a population of domestic dogs. J Vet Behav 2008;3:207–17.
56. Gazit I, Goldblatt A, Terkel J. The role of context specificity in learning: The effects of training context on explosives detection in dogs. Anim Cogn 2005;8(3):143–50.
57. Hammerle M, Horst C, Levine E, et al. 2015 AAHA canine and feline behavior management guidelines. J Am Anim Hosp Assoc 2015;51:205–21.
58. Randle H, Waran N. Breaking down barriers and dispelling myths: the need for a scientific approach to Equitation. Appl Anim Behav Sci 2017;190:1–4.
59. Veterinarian's oath. In: AVMA. Available at: https://www.avma.org/KB/Policies/Pages/veterinarians-oath.aspx. Accessed October 6, 2017.

Desensitization and Counterconditioning
When and How?

Sabrina Poggiagliolmi, DVM, MS

KEYWORDS

- Desensitization • Counterconditioning • Anxiety • Fear • Phobia

KEY POINTS

- Dogs and cats can present to a veterinary hospital because they manifest anxieties, fears, and phobias.
- These conditions can be so severe to negatively affect the patient's quality of life and the human-animal bond because some patients can become aggressive, destructive, and vocal and even hurt themselves.
- The clinician has several available tools to help the affected patient; the most implemented tools in veterinary behavioral medicine are systematic desensitization and counterconditioning.
- The goal of any desensitization and counterconditioning plan should be to make patients less or not reactive toward one or more specific triggers by learning new and more acceptable responses in their presence.

DEFINITIONS

Before proceeding with more details about the topic, it is necessary and useful to review some definitions.

Anxiety

Anxiety is a reaction of apprehension or uneasiness to an anticipated danger or threat. Signs are physiologic (autonomic arousal, increased heart and respiratory rate, trembling, salivation, gastrointestinal, and hypervigilance) and behavioral (freezing, lip licking, yawning, pacing, stress vocalizations, restlessness). Anxiety may be displayed in the absence of an identifiable stimulus. It may become generalized in some pets or may be specific to situations of perceived threat.[1]

Fear

Fear is an emotional response due to the presence or proximity of a specific stimulus (eg, object, noise, individual, social situation) that the pet perceives as a threat or

Disclosure Statement: The author has nothing to disclose.
Behavior Medicine Department, Long Island Veterinary Specialists, 163 South Service Road, Plainview, NY 11803, USA
E-mail address: spoggiagliolmi@livs.org

Vet Clin Small Anim 48 (2018) 433–442
https://doi.org/10.1016/j.cvsm.2017.12.009
vetsmall.theclinics.com

danger. It is a psychological and physiologic state characterized by somatic, emotional, cognitive, and behavioral components. It can be a normal adaptive response.[1]

Phobia

Phobia is a profound, excessive, abnormal fear response that occurs without the presence of a true threat or is out of proportion to the needs for dealing with an actual threat. Phobia is considered a maladaptive response and interferes with normal function.[1]

Desensitization

Desensitization is a behavioral treatment of phobias that involves slowly presenting the patient with increasingly strong fear-provoking stimuli while keeping the patient in a very relaxed state.[2] The more accurate wording would be *systematic desensitization*.

Counterconditioning

Counterconditioning is a negative or undesirable behavior that is extinguished or controlled by teaching the animal to do another behavior (preferably favorable and fun) that competitively interferes with the execution of the undesirable behavior.[3] For example, teaching a pet to lie down instead of jumping (the patient cannot perform both behaviors at the same time).

When desensitization and counterconditioning are implemented correctly, *response substitution* will be the end result.

Response Substitution

Response substitution is the development and exhibition of a positive desired/desired behavior or behavioral sequence that it is *incompatible* with the expression of the unwanted behavioral sequence.[4]

DESENSITIZATION AND COUNTERCONDITIONING: THE WHEN

Desensitization and counterconditioning are behavioral techniques implemented with patients that are affected by anxieties, fears, and phobias. Before starting to expose patients to any known fearful stimuli, multiple steps should be followed in order to achieve successful and enduring results (**Box 1**).[5]

Step One: Clients Compliance

Clients' compliance is an integral part of a successful plan, but it is the most difficult one to obtain and ensure, because working with pets with mental illnesses requires dedication, patience, and time, and owners tend to not to have a lot of any of the above-mentioned requirements. Owners must have realistic expectations about their pets' progress and achievements, which it is difficult to make them see and accept, because most of the time they believe their pets are simply unruly and not diseased. As Mr Benjamin Franklin rightly said, "Take time for all things: great haste makes great waste." These are words to keep in mind when we manage patients with behavioral problems.

Step Two: Having Patients Reliable on Verbal Cues

Dogs and cats do not speak English (or any other human language). Because we do not speak the same language, one way to establish clear communication with pets is through training. Clear communication should be seen as a way to convey a clear message to pets: to tell them exactly what we expect from them. Clear communication

> **Box 1**
> **Points to keep in mind to succeed in desensitization and counterconditioning**
>
> Before implementing systematic desensitization along with counterconditioning, you should be sure that the pet
>
> - Responds to verbal cues upon request;
> - Knows how to relax reliably on cue;
> - Is able to relax in its safe haven.
>
> Also, the veterinarian should assess the client's
>
> - Training skills;
> - Understanding of principles of learning;
> - Knowledge of what are their pet's favorite rewards;
> - Ability to reward their pets in a timely manner;
> - Ability to recognize signs of anxiety in their pets;
> - Availability to work at the pet's pace and not to rush the process.

can be achieved after they have learned verbal cues such as "sit," "down," "look," "touch," and other easy-to-do cues (both dogs and cats can be trained) and remind them to perform those basic behaviors upon request whenever they need or want something (**Fig. 1**). Rewarding these behaviors helps to reinforce them and provides predictability. In a sense, the pet learns how we function ("If I sit, the human gives

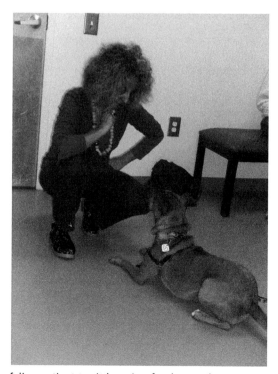

Fig. 1. Teaching a feline patient to sit by using food rewards.

me something I desire"), and in its eyes, we become predictable and extremely interesting!

Clients may need the assistance of a qualified professional dog trainer when they do not have good training skills. Veterinarians should be able to recommend trainers whose philosophy is reward based and that are familiar with the principles of learning theory.

Step Three: Learning How Pets Communicate

To better understand patients' emotional states, knowing their body language will be another important step. Pets are attuned to body language (even to our own); in fact, they communicate by using facial expressions, body postures, and vocalizations. Understanding how they use these body parts will help owners to be more aware of their pet's comfort level while being exposed to a fearful stimulus and allow them to know when to increase the intensity of the exposure accordingly. Anytime the pet will show anxiety-related signs, owners should be able to pick up on those signs and pay close attention if they are going too fast or if their pet is not comfortable yet.

The following are instructional videos about canine and feline communication, respectively:

- Zoom Room Guide to Dog Body Language (https://youtu.be/00_9JPltXHI).
- Maddie's Fund (http://www.maddiesfund.org): Feline Communication: How to Speak Cat (http://www.maddiesfund.org/feline-communication-how-to-speak-cat/presentation.html).

The following Web sites have free downloadable posters about canine and feline body language:

- Dr Sophia Yin (https://drsophiayin.com/):
  ○ Free Downloads: Posters, Handouts, and More (https://drsophiayin.com/blog/entry/free-downloads-posters-handouts-and-more/)!
- Vet Behaviour Team (http://www.vetbehaviourteam.com/):
  ○ Behavior facts sheets (http://www.vetbehaviourteam.com/client-handouts/)

Step Four: Having Good Physical Control over the Pet

Depending on the patient, there may be a need to physically control them to help them focus on the task or to prevent injuries.

Dogs may be introduced to head halters because this will allow redirecting their focus with a gentle pull of the leash, if there would be a need to. Other dogs instead must become comfortable with wearing plastic basket muzzles because it would be the only way to protect other animals and people from their unwanted biting. Basket muzzles have several advantages: they are light, they can be worn for long intervals, they allow dogs to pant, to get treats, and to drink. These are things that cloth, mesh, and neoprene muzzles do not allow.

The following Web site has educational videos on how to introduce dogs successfully to muzzles: The Muzzle up! Project (https://muzzleupproject.com/muzzle-training/).

Cats may be introduced to harnesses or to carriers; for example, both items can be extremely useful when a cat needs to be reintroduced to other household cats after having been separated because of previously aggressive encounters.

A helpful video to introduce cats to carriers can be found here:

- Catalyst Council (http://www.catalystcouncil.org/):
  ○ Cats & Carriers: Friends not Foes (https://youtu.be/9RGY5oSKVfo).

Step Five: Medications and/or Natural Supplements

Some patients are so distressed that they cannot focus on any training, not even on very easy tasks, and cannot start desensitization and counterconditioning to stimuli. This is when medications and/or natural supplements should be considered and recommended: they will help to make the patient more comfortable in its own skin because they stabilize the patient's mood.

Pheromones (there is no unanimous consent[6–8]) and essential oils[9] (eg, lavender) may have a calming effect as well. Playing classical music[10] or white noise may help to distract the patient from fear-evoking stimuli.

Clients should be warned that there is no "magic bullet" in veterinary behavioral medicine. Medications and natural supplements are just one of the many tools that are available to manage patients' problems. They should never be given alone, but in combination with a behavior modification treatment plan to guarantee more favorable outcomes. Just relying on medications will set that patient up for failure, and it will just add more stress to the owner's frustration because no definitive change in the pet's behavior will be noticed. Additional information on medications and behavioral diets can be found in the Leslie Sinn article, "Advances in Behavioral Psychopharmacology;" and Jillian M. Orlando author, "Behavioral Nutraceuticals and Diets," of this issue.

Step Six: Choose the Pet Favorite Reward

When we train pets, we should give them a valid motivation for working. Obviously, because they are not human beings, they cannot be paid with money, but they will work for rewards. Rewards must be seen as a salary, which is given when the pet has done a good job (eg, complying with our requests). A reward is anything the pet likes (food, praises, play time, toys), but not necessarily the owner. For example, some owners are hesitant or against the use of food as a reward because they feel that it is used more as a bribe and not as a "compensation" for a job well done. It should be explained to the owners that the reward will be given only after the behavior is performed (and only if it will be performed) and not before or for free. Usually, this should help to clarify the misconception.

Step Seven: Teaching Pets How to Relax

It is essential for any patient to be able to relax because no learning can be achieved if the patient is anxious or scared. There are several protocols for relaxation[11–13] that can be found in any of the available veterinary behavioral medicine textbooks. Their main goal is to teach the patient to relax preferably on a mat (or any other comfortable spot). Once the patient has mastered the exercise, clients will be able to send the patient to that designated safe haven to relax; the pet can seek out the space on his own as well (**Fig. 2**).

The patient will learn to stay relaxed and remain in its spot while being distracted: the distractions to which the pet will be exposed will gradually become more complicated. The intent is to teach the pet that whatever happens around them, there is no need to freak out, because only good things will surround them (eg, getting their favorite treat or toy).

The layout of one of the relaxation protocol is provided in **Box 2**.

Step Eight: Avoid Punishment

Punishment should be avoided because the pet is not acting out of spite or dominance, but out of fear. Reprimanding a phobic pet will make that pet even more anxious because it would associate the scary event with a painful and unpleasant

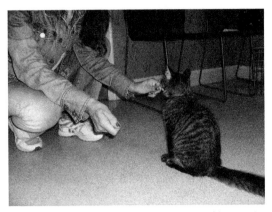

Fig. 2. The author practicing relaxation exercises with one of her patients.

experience as well. This can be dangerous in cases of fear-based aggression toward people and animals.

DESENSITIZATION AND COUNTERCONDITIONING: THE HOW

Once the patient is deemed ready to starting desensitization and counterconditioning, a stimulus gradient must be determined, meaning that once a stimulus has been identified, it will be necessary to make a list starting from the least scary component of that stimulus to the scariest one. The list is crucial because it provides a structure for the therapy. Exposures should start with a muted stimulus. For example, if a pet is scared of storms, the first exposure will start with a recording of light rain and not of a loud thunder.

Using a stimulus gradient prevents the development of another phenomenon: sensitization (an increased response to a repeated stimulus) and the opposite of our goal.

HOW: EXAMPLE 1: TREATING DOGS WITH NOISE PHOBIAS

Dogs affected by noise sensitivities are a common occurrence in any veterinary hospital. If you have a patient that is scared when it hears a clap of thunder, your main goal is to make this dog less scared of this loud rumbling noise. Ideally, the training session should take place on a sunny day or a long time before the start of the storm season. Sessions should not be longer than 5 to 10 minutes, and they can be repeated multiple times a day. The patient should reliably go to his place and relax when prompted.

Different CDs are available on the market to desensitize dogs to loud noises; examples of CDs that can be acquired by clients are the following:

- Canine Noise Phobia: Thunderstorms, CD (https://icalmpet.com/product/canine-noise-phobias-thunderstorms/).
- Sounds Good CD–Thunderstorms (http://216.119.127.16/store/index.php?p=product&id=10&parent=2).

The CD is played at the lowest volume possible while the dog relaxes on its mat. Please note that the dog's sense of hearing is definitely better than ours and that what we intend for low volume may be already too high for the dog. The dog should be kept busy with a favored and special reward. Special means that the chosen reward is kept away except during training sessions. The main reason for doing this is to keep the dog's interest in that reward high by not making it available 24/7.

Box 2
Example of a relaxation protocol

Tranquility Training Exercises

Listed are guidelines for a series of daily training exercises, taking less than 10 minutes to complete. These guidelines are the foundation for later desensitization and counterconditioning exercises. It may be more successful to start with the dog on leash and head collar and then progress to off-leash training on the second rotation through the exercises. If the dog's problematic behaviors only occur outside the home, do all the tranquility training on leash. If a dog routinely gets bored, distracted, agitated, or distressed during these exercises, they can be broken down into two 5-minute sessions. The person with the most control over the pet should begin the training first.

- Find a quiet place in your home for initial training.
- In some cases, you may want to use a small rug or bed as a location to train your pet to settle and relax.
  - Using a rug or bed will allow you to take this item to other locations where your pet may need to be calm. Naturally, if the problem occurs outdoors, this is not necessary.
  - Having a reliable "go to X" command is very helpful for a wide range of undesirable behaviors ranging from obnoxious greeting behaviors to aggression.
  - This can be used in separation anxiety exercises for independence training and teaching a safe place to remain when alone.
- In all of the exercises, the dog has to do a simple command (sit or down) and then remain in that position and in a tranquil state to gain the reward.
- You may want to add in a key phrase like "relax" or "easy" to teach the dog to associate relaxation with sit/down and stay.
  - The goal is for the pet to be relaxed and calm.
  - Relaxation is measured by watching the facial expressions and body postures of your pet; ears should be relaxed and the body soft and loose.
  - You also want slow and relaxed respirations.
- As you progress through the exercises, the handler will start to engage in mild distractions during the command phase.
- Remember that the handler throughout the exercise should give the dog verbal direction. The distractions will become greater as the training progresses.
- Noncompliance is not rewarded. Just turn away, take a short (eg, 30-s) break, and adjust the exercise to increase chances of success and then try again.
- Between each exercise, the dog should break the sit, get up and move, and sit again. To get this to happen, the handler can move to another spot in the room and call the dog to them for the next exercise.
- The first round of these exercises should be done inside the house with minimal household distractions; other dogs should be confined elsewhere, and it should be quiet, and so forth.
- The second round can be in slightly more distracting circumstances, such as in a secure yard.
- Once the dog has successfully completed these exercises in at least 2 different locations, you can progress to desensitization and counterconditioning to the trigger stimuli.

Example Training Day

Day One

1. Sit

2. Sit; watch you for 2 seconds

3. Sit; watch you for 5 seconds

4. Release for a rest 5. Go to spot; sit

6. Sit; watch you for 3 seconds

7. Sit; watch you while you take one step backwards and return

8. Release for a rest

9. Go to spot; sit; stay for 3 seconds

10. Sit; watch you while you raise your free arm to chest level and return it to your side again

11. Go to spot; sit; watch you for 10 seconds

12. Sit while you walk one step to the right and return

13. Go to spot; sit while you walk 2 steps backward and return

14. Sit; watch you for 5 seconds

15. Go to spot; sit while you walk 3 steps backward and return

16. Sit; watch you for 5 seconds

Day Two

1. Repeat steps 1 to 16, varying the time the pet remains in place from 3 to 10 seconds

2. Vary the direction of movement; go left, then back, swivel, and turn away one step and return, or turn in a circle or march in place

3. Vary the distraction, perhaps clapping your hands softly 2 to 3 times

Subsequent Days

1. For the remainder of the first week, continue to vary the amount of time the pet remains stationary in each step

2. Continue to vary the distractions, include jumping jacks, knocking on furniture, talking, jogging in place, turning your back on the dog, and so forth

3. After a week, return to day one and repeat in a different location

4. Repeat with different family members handling the pet

From Horwitz DF, Neilson JC. Tranquility training exercises. In: Horwitz DF, Neilson JC, editors. Blackwell's five minute veterinary consult clinical companion canine & feline behavior. Ames (IA): Blackwell Publishing; 2007. p. 576–7; with permission.

In the meantime, the owner must monitor closely the dog response to the CD. The dog's body language should indicate relaxation. If at any moment the dog shows signs of fear, the session should be terminated and ended on a positive note.

Over time, the volume of the CD will be increased according to the body language of the dog. If done properly, eventually the CD will be played at full volume with the dog not being affected minimally by it.

HOW: EXAMPLE 2: TREATING CATS WITH FEAR OF PEOPLE

Initially, the cat should be confined in a room behind a closed door because it needs to know that it has a safe haven, a place to hide and feel at ease while it is kept away from the scary unfamiliar person. Comfortable beddings, water and food bowls, and favorite toys should be available to the cat. Owners should be able to distract their pets and practice some relaxation exercises or training, play with them, or offer them their favorite treats in exchange for more relaxed body postures while the stranger is on the other side of the door. Gradually and over days, the cat may be fed closer and closer to the door until it will regularly eat by it when the person stays quietly on the other side. Obviously, the speed at which the desensitization and counterconditioning process takes place depends on the cat's body language: as soon as signs of anxiety are noticed, the unfamiliar person should move away from the door. The next exposure should start at the most distant point from the door where the cat felt more relaxed. When the cat will accept the presence of the person by the door without showing any sign of aggression, the door may be cracked open so that the cat can see the person. The person can start tossing treats at the cat's direction, and if the cat will accept them, the person can ask the cat to sit before rewarding it with the next treat. When the door can be left completely open because the cat is calm and relaxed, it is important that the person refrains from touching the cat because this approach may backfire. Instead, the cat should be left free to investigate its surroundings, and anytime it will show interest toward the person, it will be rewarded with its favorite treats (preferred food is reserved only for training sessions). If the cat has been introduced to a harness, this will be the perfect time to have the cat wear it with a leash attached to it: in the case of a fearful reaction, the cat may be safely removed from the situation and moved back into his room without anyone being hurt.

If the cat's pace is respected, the cat will eventually accept unfamiliar people, because it has had enough time to learn that they are a predictor of pleasant experiences and encounters because nothing stressful happens when they are in the house.

SUMMARY

Desensitization and counterconditioning are extremely useful techniques that can help our patients overcome their anxieties and fears, but the techniques need to be followed carefully in order to see and maintain long-lasting results.

REFERENCES

1. Landsberg G, Hunthausen W, Ackerman L. Fears, phobias, and anxiety disorders. In: Landsberg G, Hunthausen W, Ackerman L, editors. Behavior problems of the dog & cat. 3rd edition. Cambridge (United Kingdom): Elsevier; 2013. p. 182.
2. Mazur EM. Glossary. In: Mazur EM, editor. Learning and behavior. 7th edition. Upper Saddle River (NJ): Pearson; 2013. p. 334.
3. Overall KL. Treatment of behavioral problems. In: Overall KL, editor. Clinical behavioral medicine for small animals. St Louis (MO): Mosby; 1997. p. 277.
4. Overall KL. Changing behavior: roles for learning, negotiated settlements, and individualized treatment plans. In: Overall KL, editor. Manual of clinical behavioral medicine for dogs and cats. St Louis (MO): Mosby; 2013. p. 74.
5. Horwitz DF, Neilson JC. Desensitization and counterconditioning: the details. In: Horwitz DF, Neilson JC, editors. Blackwell's five minute veterinary consult clinical companion canine & feline behavior. Ames (IA): Blackwell Publishing; 2007. p. 554–5.
6. Frank D, Beauchamp G, Palestrini C. Systematic review of the use of pheromones for treatment of undesirable behavior in cats and dogs. J Am Vet Med Assoc 2010;236(12):1308–16.
7. Chadwin RM, Bain MJ, Kass PH. Effect of a synthetic feline facial pheromone product on stress scores and incidence of upper respiratory tract infection in shelter cats. J Am Vet Med Assoc 2017;251(4):413–20.
8. Conti LMC, Champion T, Guberman UC, et al. Evaluation of environment and a feline facial pheromone analogue on physiologic and behavioral measures in cats. J Feline Med Surg 2017;19(2):165–70.

9. Wells DL. Aromatherapy for travel-induced excitement in dogs. J Am Vet Med Assoc 2006;229(6):964-7.

10. Kogan LR, Schoenfeld-Tacher R, Simon AA. Behavioral effects of auditory stimulation on kenneled dogs. J Vet Behav 2012;7:268-75.

11. Horwitz DF, Neilson JC. Tranquility training exercises. In: Horwitz DF, Neilson JC, editors. Blackwell's five minute veterinary consult clinical companion canine & feline behavior. Ames (IA): Blackwell Publishing; 2007. p. 576-7.

12. Overall KL. Protocol for relaxation: behavior modification tier 1. In: Overall KL, editor. Manual of clinical behavioral medicine for dogs and cats. St Louis (MO): Mosby; 2013. p. 585-98.

13. Landsberg G, Hunthausen W, Ackerman L. Treatment – behavior modification techniques. In: Landsberg G, Hunthausen W, Ackerman L, editors. Behavior problems of the dog & cat. 3rd edition. Cambridge (United Kingdom): Elsevier; 2013. p. 110-1.

Special Considerations for Diagnosing Behavior Problems in Older Pets

Eranda Rajapaksha, BVSc, MS, PhD

KEYWORDS

- Behavior • Cognitive dysfunction syndrome • Aging • Older pets

KEY POINTS

- Aging is a complex process that involves changes in sensory perception, cognition, and physical strength. These changes can lead to age-related behavior problems.
- Cognitive dysfunction syndrome is a progressive neurodegenerative disease in older dogs and cats. Affected pets show typical behavioral changes.
- It is difficult to diagnose behavioral problems in older pets because first signs of many underlying degenerative disease conditions are reflected as a behavioral change.
- Proper history taking, general clinical examination, laboratory examination, and consideration of cognitive dysfunction syndrome signs are important steps in diagnosis.
- A combination of client education, behavioral and environmental enrichment, balanced nutrition, and pharmacologic intervention improves the behavioral problems and quality of life in an aging pet.

INTRODUCTION

Pet animals in modern society live longer than their ancestors due to improved nutrition and health care. Life expectancy in dogs doubled during past 4 decades and house cats live twice the age of their wild counterparts.[1] The average life span of domestic dog varies from 6.7 years to 12 years and smaller dog breeds tend to live longer.[2] It is thought that increased hormonal activities, such as insulin-like growth factor 1, and faster growth rate in larger breeds, make their bodies more susceptible to disease and accelerate the aging process. Age calculation in pet animals varies according to the species and breed. Small breed dogs are considered geriatric at the age of 7 years whereas dogs of larger breeds are considered geriatric when they are 6 years of age.[1] Cats are considered geriatric at 7 years to 11 years of age. In general, a pet is considered geriatric when the animal is in the last 25% of the life span predicted for its breed.[3]

The author has nothing to disclose.
Veterinary Clinical Sciences, University of Peradeniya, Peradeniya 20400, Sri Lanka
E-mail address: earajapaksha@gmail.com

Vet Clin Small Anim 48 (2018) 443–456
https://doi.org/10.1016/j.cvsm.2017.12.010

Effects of Aging in a Pet

Effects of aging can lead to medical issues like neoplasia, cardiovascular disease, kidney/urinary tract disease, liver disease, diabetes, joint/bone disease, and weakness in older pets. Behavioral changes may be an early indicator of these conditions. In addition to these medical changes, behavioral problems, such as separation anxiety, human-directed/intraspecies aggression, house soiling, excessive vocalization, phobias, sleep-wake cycle alteration, aimless or repetitive behaviors, reduced self-hygiene, and decreased responsiveness to stimuli can be observed in older pets.[3,4]

Human and Companion Animal Bond

Emotional attachment plays an important role in the relationship between humans and the pet animals.[5] Due to the long history of canine domestication and adaptation to the human environment, dogs and their owners have special attachments similar to a human parent-offspring attachment, where the animal is dependent on the caregiver.[6] Therefore, the nature of the relationship between owner and pet can have a significant impact on an animal's quality of life. It is shown that puppies form an attachment with their owners as young as 16 weeks of age and studies conducted in shelters showed that even the socially deprived adult dogs tend to form attachments with their handlers.[7,8] This attachment behavior in dogs is thought to be due to genetic selection that occurred in the course of domestication. Even though several studies have been conducted on the attachment of puppies and young adults with humans, there is not much research conducted on the attachment of older dogs and how the human-dog attachment changes with the aging of both pet and owner. Physiologic changes during the aging process, especially decreased sensory perception, can have a significant effect on the attachment between an older dog and owner. This change can be reflected as a behavioral change in an aging dog. Older dogs (more than 7 years of age) have shown increased stress response when they are exposed to a new environment or when separated from the owners.[5]

CAUSES OF BEHAVIORAL CHANGES IN OLDER PETS

Due to the physical, metabolic, and emotional changes of the aging process, older pets tend to have more behavioral problems than younger pets, and causes of most of these problems also are different from those of younger pets (**Box 1**).

Medical Conditions

Behavioral change in an older pet might be the first indicator of an irreversible degenerative condition in the animal. In particular, painful conditions, such as osteoarthritis, neoplasias, encephalopathies, and dental diseases, can lead to increased aggression or

---

Box 1
Major causes of behavioral problems observed in older pets

1. Medical conditions
2. Age-related behavioral changes
3. Stress-related behaviors
4. Multiple intersecting factors
5. Primary (nonmedical) behavioral problems
6. CDS

decreased social interactions. Endocrinopathies, cataracts, and deafness can show profound changes in the way a pet interacts with its environment. Activity level, elimination pattern, and the sleep-wake cycle of an old pet can be affected by diseases in the renal, cardiac, and gastrointestinal systems. Systemic medical conditions that occur with the age and behavioral changes in the pets are shown in **Table 1**. Neoplastic processes are not included because most of them spread to several systems and the behavior changes vary with the type of tumor. Tumors in the bone, central nervous system, gastrointestinal system, prostate, mammary gland, and intranasal, intrathoracic, abdominal, oral, and pharyngeal areas are frequently associated with pain and pain-related behaviors, such as aggression, irritability, declined social interaction, and vocalization, seen in affected pets.[29] Infectious disease, such as feline immunodeficiency virus, feline leukemia virus, and toxoplasmosis, can also cause behavioral changes in cats.[30]

Common Age-Related Behavioral Changes

Normal degeneration in muscles and organ systems, lack of energy reserves in the aging body, and gradual loss of adaptive capacity can be reflected as behavioral changes in an aging pet, separate and distinct from specific medical pathologies. Lethargy, decreased appetite, decreased activity, and reduced frequency of oral activities, such as licking or nibbling, in an older pet can be features of a normal aging process.[31]

Stress-Related Behaviors

Stress due to changes in the human-animal bond or the environmental or owner schedule change can affect the behavior of a pet. Older pets can have prominent behavioral changes due to stress because adaptation to stressful situations declines with the aging. Changes in regular activity, sleep-wake cycle, and social interaction; reduced water and/or feed intake; and increased huddling or shivering are common stress-related behavior changes noted by pet owners. Similarly, vocalization, aggression or apathy, increased sensitivity, depression, house soiling, decreased play, phobia, and separation anxiety are some prominent behavioral changes associated with stress in pet animals of all ages.[32] In addition to the behavioral signs there can be physiologic changes, such as increased heart rate, panting, salivation, and dilated pupils in a stressed animal and in most cases go un-noticed by clients.

The Effect of Multiple Intersecting Factors

Older pets tend to have multiple medical conditions and, either alone or in combination with environment, stress, and other factors, these conditions can give rise to behavioral problems. As an example, a dog suffering from osteoarthritis and deafness can become more aggressive compared with an animal with only one of these conditions. Also, some behavioral problems that were ignored by an owner become prominent and nontolerable when combined with a disease condition. As an example, house soiling in a poorly trained pet can become an exacerbated problem if an animal has a renal disease.

Primary (Nonmedical) Behavioral Problems

Due to a lower threshold level for tolerating social or environmental change, older pets can more easily develop primary behavioral problems than when they were young. Changes, such as moving to a new house, loss of a household member (person or a pet), schedule change, and addition of a new member to the house (person or a new pet), are more likely to trigger onset of a behavior issue in an older than a younger pet. Therefore, primary behavior problems, such as aggression, anxiety, and fear-based conditions and phobias, could develop as pets get older.

Table 1
Common systemic medical conditions in older pets and observed behavior changes

Body System	Condition	Behavioral Change
Musculoskeletal	Osteoarthritis[9]	Reduced mobility and stiffness, irritability, altered gait, reluctance to go up or down stairs, aggression, house soiling, decreased activity, decreased social interaction, attention seeking, aggression, whimpering
	Obesity[10]	Reduced activity, lethargy
	Weight loss[11]	Lethargy, exercise intolerance, irritability, food-seeking (if polyphagic), aggression (if due to pain or neoplasm), avoidance of food, selective eating, anorexic, pica, night waking, house soiling
Gastrointestinal	Inflammatory bowel disease[3]	Decreased appetite, selective eating, reduced activity, restlessness, changing positions, irritability, house soiling, night waking, lip licking, pica
	Constipation[3]	Decreased appetite, straining, irritability and discomfort, house soiling
	Decreased hepatic function[3]	Loss of appetite, weight loss, polyuria, polydipsia, abnormal gait, weakness, confusion, seizures, if brain is affected can show nervous signs of hepatic encephalopathy
	Periodontal disease[12]/tooth resorption[13]	Aggression, irritability, loss of interest in food, vocalizing, head shyness
Endocrine	Hyperthyroidism in cats[14]	Polyphagia, polyuria, polydipsia, hyperactivity, irritability, aggression, increased appetite and vocalization
	Hypothyroidism in dogs[15]	Lethargy, mental dullness, sluggishness, disorientation, circling
	Hyperadrenocorticism[15]	Panting, polyphagia, polyuria, polydipsia, restlessness, altered elimination habits
	Hyperparathyroidism[15]	Polyuria, polydipsia, lethargy, house soiling, anxiety
	Diabetes mellitus[15,16]	Polyuria, polydipsia, house soiling, polyphagia
Central nervous system	Spinal cord disease and/or peripheral neuropathies[3]	scratching motion without touching the skin, self-mutilation, increased frequency in looking at the same area, yelping, decreased activity and appetite, aggression
Sensory	Cataract, retinal disease, keratoconjunctivitis sicca[3]	Decreased response, changes in sleep-wake cycle, decreed ability to perform normal daily activities, disorientation, confusion
Body system	Condition	Behavioral change

(continued on next page)

Table 1 (continued)		
Body System	Condition	Behavioral Change
Sensory	Deafness[3]	Decreased/altered response to stimuli, sometimes more reactive and sensitive (to touch), anxious, disorientation
Urinary	Chronic renal failure[17]	Polyuria, polydipsia, nocturia, anorexia, selective eating, irritability and nervous signs if uremic
	Urinary tract infection[17] Nephrolithiasis[17]	House soiling, urine spaying, irritability
Reproduction	Prostatic disease[3]	House soiling, irritability, lethargy
Cardiovascular system	Myocardial fibrosis[18]/valvular fibrocalcification,[18] chronic valvular disease[19]/pericardial disease[19]/arrhythmia[19]/ hypertension[20]/cardiomyopathy[20]/ arteriosclerosis[21]	Lethargy, syncope, anorexia, exercise intolerance
Hematopoietic	Anemia[3]	Lethargy, exercise intolerance, panting
Immune	Leukopenia[22]	Lethargy, decreased appetite, irritability
Dermatologic	Skin and subcutaneous masses[3]	Increased irritability, licking, self-mutilation, increased sensitivity
Respiratory	Chronic rhinitis[3]/chronic bronchitis[3]/ decrease chest wall compliance[23]/ tracheal collapse[3]/laryngeal paralysis[3]	Exercise intolerance, panting, decreased activity

A Special Diagnosis: Cognitive Dysfunction Syndrome

Cognitive dysfunction syndrome (CDS) is a widely documented behavior condition in older dogs and cats. This is often listed as separate behavior diagnosis although many clinical signs are common to what is presented with primary behavior problems. CDS is a progressive neurodegenerative disease in older dogs and cats. It is thought to be a pathologic aging process due to oxidative stress and other structural changes in the brain.[33] Several microscopic and macroscopic changes are identified in brains of older dogs and cats with CDS[34]; these include the deposition of β-amyloid plaques in the hippocampus and cerebral cortex and perivascular changes, including arteriosclerosis and infarcts.

Affected pets show typical behavioral changes that are summarized by the acronym DISHA[32]: spatial Disorientation (including "getting lost" in the house or yard or "stuck" behind furniture), alteration in social Interactions (perhaps not seeming to recognize owners), Sleep-wake cycle disturbance, House soiling, and changes in Activity are these typical behaviors.[35] Loss of house-training and sleep-wake disturbances are particularly difficult for pet owners. Changes in activity can be reflected as an increased or repetitive action, decreased activity, or depression-related and anxiety-related behaviors. Affected service dogs and animals that are trained for specific tasks might show decline in memory function and learning ability.[36] Inappropriate vocalization, especially during the night, and decreased self-hygiene are also 2 prominent signs of CDS in cats.[37]

DIAGNOSIS OF BEHAVIORAL PROBLEMS IN OLDER PETS

Aging is a complex process that involves changes in sensory perception, cognition, and physical strength of an animal. These changes can lead to age-related behavior problems. In addition, systemic diseases or environment change can elicit a behavioral change in an old dog or a cat. Therefore, it is challenging to diagnose age-related behavioral problems.

Separation anxiety, human-directed aggression, house soiling, vocalization, and phobias are the most common behavioral problems in older dogs.[4] House soiling and excessive vocalization are the most common problems in older cats.[4,37] These common behavioral problems are also indicative of many underlying disease conditions. Therefore, it is essential to perform a thorough clinical and laboratory examination to screen the pets for other medical problems before focusing on a primary behavioral problem. Detailed history taking also plays an important role because certain medications, such as steroids, can have potential behavior effects, such as nervousness, restlessness, startle response, food guarding, irritable aggression, and increased avoidance response.[38]

Fig. 1 illustrates the clinical steps to be taken when an older pet is presented for a problem behavior. Detailed history taking and general clinical examination are essential processes in the diagnosis. General clinical examination should include weight, body condition score, blood pressure measurement to diagnose hypertension, neurologic examination, and sensory examination for vision and hearing. Blood and urine samples need to be collected for laboratory testing. Complete blood cell count, serum biochemistry, urinalysis, and thyroid profile are the laboratory tests that may be of value in a geriatric patient. If needed, further radiographic, ultrasound, or serologic tests can be conducted to confirm a disease condition. If a medical condition is not detected, a behavior examination can be conducted to rule out CDS. Landsberg and colleagues[36] provide a checklist that can be used in questioning the owner and assessing the behavior of pets. If there are positive signs of CDS, then further confirmatory tests, such as the oddity discrimination task[39] and delayed-nonmatching to position task,[40] can be performed. If the CDS behavioral signs are not present in the animal, a detailed behavioral evaluation needs to be performed on the pet. Results of the behavioral examination, general clinical examination findings (signs of stress, such as dilated pupil, panting, and salivation) and facts obtained during history taking (change in environment or social interaction, medication, and exposure to a toxin) need to be considered in the final diagnosis of a behavioral problem.

DEVELOPMENT OF A TREATMENT AND MANAGEMENT PLAN

Irrespective of age, treatment of behavior problems requires multimodal therapeutic approaches. Customized behavior modification plans, environmental changes, pharmacologic interventions, and detailed client awareness are important aspects of a successful treatment plan. Therefore, treatment can be broadly separated in to counseling for clients, nonpharmacologic strategies, and pharmacologic strategies.

Managing Expectations and Counseling Clients

When treating older pets, it is important to help client understand that their pet has reached a state where the level and type of interactions need alterations. It is not uncommon for clients to expect the vigor and response of a younger animal in their old pet. Young children, in particular, who have grown up with pets, tend to think of a pet's age in terms of human years. Therefore, it is important to make them aware that the pet has reached the last quarter of life and that irreversible physiologic changes occur with the aging process. This helps owners adjust their interaction and improve the

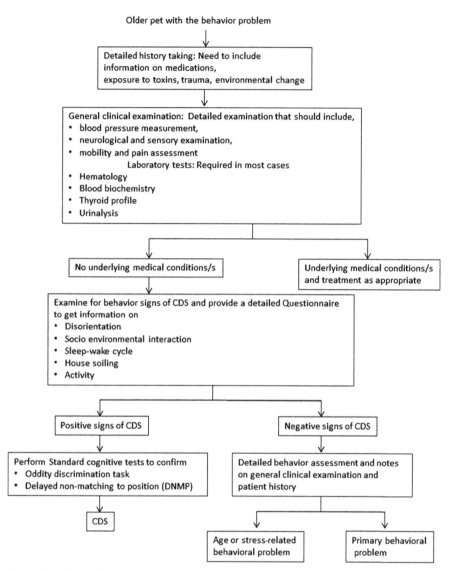

Fig. 1. Flow chart illustrating the steps to be taken when diagnosing a behavioral problem in older pets.

relationship with the pet. Making owners aware of age-associated diseases and behavioral changes is important for early detection of medical or behavioral issues in aging pet. This makes for easier disease management, better quality of life for pets.

Nonpharmacologic Strategies

Improving quality of life by behavioral and environmental modifications

Both behavioral and environmental modifications should focus on stimulating mental activity and altering daily behavioral time budget of the pets to match their physical abilities. Studies have shown that stimulation of canine brain activity is an integral element in maintaining quality of life for older pets.[41] These modifications can include gentle play, training, tolerable exercise, and introduction of novel toys. Activities and tasks should match the capabilities of the pet and should be able to stimulate learning and memory in patients with cognitive dysfunction. Older pets may not tolerate inconsistencies in their daily activities due to stress involved with life changes.[32] Therefore the environmental changes need to be gradual and pets need to be given enough time to adapt and choose their preferences. Detailed feedback with clients is important for the success of behavioral and environmental modification.

Added enrichments enhance the positive social interactions in pets. Aging pets that show social detachments can benefit from exploration, hunt, search, and retrieve activities as well as interactive training sessions with owners. Food toys and play that involve limb-eye coordination are physically and mentally stimulating. Products containing dog-appeasing pheromone, feline facial pheromone, and catnip can be helpful in attracting pets to initiate play.

Changing the physical environment and routine activities can help older pets cope with their behavior problems. Dogs with house-soiling problems due to increased urine frequency may benefit from frequent trips outdoors or by addition of an indoor toilet area. In cats, inappropriate elimination due to litterbox aversion can be improved by providing more litter boxes with nonslip ramps that reduce pain associated with elimination. Ramps, carts, and trolleys can be introduced to pets living with pain and discomfort at locomotion to improve mobility with minimum discomfort.

Night-time sleeplessness in an aging pet can potentially be addressed by management of the pet's day-night cycle. Access to daylight during the day and reduced exposure to artificial light at night, along with increased daytime enrichment play sessions prior to bed, can help pets sleep better at night.

Nutritional and dietary management

Nutritional balance and dietary adjustments can help older pets reduce the effects of aging. Free radicals play a key role in brain aging and development of CDS. Their negative effects of can be reduced by antioxidant supplements in the diet.[42,43] Docosahexaenoic acid (DHA) is required for efficient neuronal function and studies have shown a decrease in DHA in the aging brain. Supplementation of DHA in the form of fish oil might be beneficial for older pets with CDS. Providing an alternative energy source other than glucose also is beneficial because there is a decrease in glucose metabolism efficiency with aging.[44] Lactates, ketone bodies, and fatty acids derived from medium-chain triglycerides are some alternative energy sources included in geriatric diets.[11]

Currently available commercial diets for older pets mainly focus in delaying cognitive decline and can be prescribed in dogs with CDS. Nutritional trials have shown improvement in performing cognitive tasks in dogs given diets containing broad-spectrum antioxidants and mitochondrial enzymatic cofactors[43] and dogs given supplementation with medium-chain triglycerides.[44] It is also shown that the greatest benefit is obtained by diet in combination with environmental enrichment.[42] There are no published studies on dietary improvement of brain function in cats and it is recommended to provide antioxidants and omega-3-fatty acids for aging cats (see Jillian M. Orlando's article, "Behavioral Nutraceuticals and Diets," in this issue, for information on particular diets).

Nutraceuticals and supplements

A range of nutraceuticals and supplements is in the market place for geriatric pets and most are used for cognitive enhancement. A detailed list of these products and their dosages is documented by Lansberg and colleagues.[36] These products contain phospholipids, fatty acids, antioxidants, herbal extracts, vitamins, and mitochondrial cofactors. Some commonly used commercial nutraceuticals and their potential benefits are listed in **Table 2**. Of these products, Senilife (Ceva Animal Health, Lenexa, KS) is labeled for both cats and dogs although efficacy is not tested in cats. Similarly, the feline version of Aktivait (VetPlus, Lancashire, England) is yet to be tested in clinical trials. Novifit (Virbac, Fort Worth, TX), a product containing S-adenosyl-L-methionine (SAMe), has been tested as effective in both cats and dogs but caution is needed when combined with drugs that increase serotonin, because SAMe can increase central serotonin levels. In general, the use of nutraceuticals and supplements should be done with caution and it is recommended to have regular laboratory profiles of pets that are subjected to long-term use.

Pharmacologic Strategies for Treatment of Behavior Problems in Older Pets

Older pets with primary behavior problems can benefit by pharmacologic interventions in conjunction with behavior modification plan. Detailed pharmacologic strategies for primary behavior problems in dogs and cats are given in other articles (see Leslie Sinn article, "Advances in Behavioral Psychopharmacology," in this issue); the main focus of this section is on CDS. One important point in CDS is that it cannot be cured but progression of the clinical signs and decline in cognitive function can be delayed—or temporarily reversed—with medication. When prescribing for old age pets, it is important for practitioners to be mindful of physiologic changes that come with advanced age. Some other important factors to be considered when prescribing for a pet are given in **Box 2**.

Several drugs are available to improve and control the clinical signs of CDS in dogs. A summary on dosage and the mode of action of the most commonly used drugs is given in **Table 3**. There are no licensed medications to treat cats for CDS.

Selegiline (Anipryl; Pfizer Animal Health, New York, New York), which is only licensed for dogs, has shown improvement with CDS both clinically and in controlled laboratory experiments. It is suggested that selegiline may enhance dopamine and other catecholamines in the brain and may also act as a neuroprotective agent by acting on oxygen free radicals.[45,47] Off-label use of selegiline in cats has also shown improvement in CDS-like signs.[48] Selegiline should not be prescribed for patients using other monoamine oxidase inhibitors, such as Amitraz, and caution should be used with concurrent use with drugs that increase serotonin transmission. Therefore, concurrent use of

Table 2	
Commonly used nutraceuticals and their effects in older pets	
Name of Nutraceutical	**Effect on Older Pet**
Senilife; Ceva Animal Health, Libourne, France	Improved memory performance[24]—for both dogs and cats
Aktivait; VetPlus Ltd, Lytham St. Annes, UK	Improvement in signs of disorientation, social interactions, and house soiling[25]—for dogs
Novifit; Virbac, Fort Worth, TX	Improvement in activity and awareness[26]—for dogs and cats
Neutricks; Quincy Animal Health, Madison, WI	Improved learning and attention[27]—for dogs
Cholodin-FEL; MVP Laboratories, Omaha, NE	Improvement in confusion and appetite[28]—for cats

See Jillian M. Orlando article, "Behavioral Nutraceuticals and Diets," in this issue, for information on nutraceuticals.

Box 2
Important points to be considered by veterinary practitioners during pharmacologic interventions

- Both veterinarian and client should understand that use of medication is only 1 element of the behavioral management and treatment plan.
- Except the few products that are—or have been—licensed for use in dogs, such as fluoxetine, clomipramine, dexmedetomidine, and selegiline, many medications are yet to be assessed for pharmacologic properties in pets.
- Widespread species and individual variations need to be considered and veterinarians should plan to reach sufficient therapeutic effect with minimum adverse effects by titrating from lower end of the dose up to the maximum.
- Contraindications and drug interactions need to be considered and referring veterinarians and clients should be kept informed.
- Minimum database of the patient, including a complete blood cell count, serum biochemistry values, and urinalysis, needs to be investigated before prescription of medication and this should always be followed for off-label medications.

---

selective serotonin reuptake inhibitors, tricyclic antidepressants, buspirone, trazodone, tramadol, and dextromethorphan should be done cautiously or avoided.

Propentofylline (Vivitonin; MSD Animal Health, Milton Keynes, United Kingdom) can be used to treat lethargic and depressed dogs and effects may be due to increase blood flow to the muscles and brain. Use of propentofylline has been documented in dogs, but behavioral changes in dogs and clinical of efficacy in cats is not yet proved in clinical trials.[49]

Nicergoline is licensed in some countries to help dogs with age-related behavior disorders. This is an α_1-adrenergic and α_2-adrenergic that may increase cerebral blood flow, inhibit platelet aggregation, and enhance neuronal transmission.[46]

Table 3
Dosage and mode of action of most commonly used drugs to treat cognitive dysfunction syndrome

Drug and Dosages	Mode of action	Points to Remember
Selegiline Dog: 0.5–1 mg/kg sid in the morning Cat: 0.5–1 mg/kg sid in the morning	Selective and irreversible inhibitor of monoamine oxidase B.[45]	• May require 2 wk or longer before improvement • Not to be prescribed with other monoamine oxidase inhibitors • Be cautious in concurrent use with drugs that increase serotonin transmission.
Propentofylline Dog: 2.5–5 mg/kg bid Cat: $^1/_4$ of 50-mg tablet daily	Inhibit uptake of adenosine and blocking phosphodiesterase[46]	• Licensed in some European countries • Testing has been limited to clinical trials.
Nicergoline Dog: 0.25–0.5 mg/kg sid in the morning Cat: suggested dose, $^1/_4$ of 5 mg q24h	Increase dopamine and noradrenaline turnover[46]	• Licensed in some countries

Adrafinil and modafinil can improve alertness in older dogs. These medications stimulate noradrenergic system and also help in maintaining normal sleep-wake cycles by promoting daytime locomotor activity in dogs.[50,51] Dosage and efficacy of these drugs need to be established in older dogs. Adrafinil have shown to increase locomotion and enhance learning while showing memory impairment.[51] This raises a concern of improving one function at the cost of another in the treatment plan. Therefore, use of this drug needs careful attention.

Other pharmacologic drugs that have been used and discussed in older pets are cholinesterase inhibitors, nonsteroidal anti-inflammatory drugs, statins, N-methyl-D-aspartate receptor antagonists, and hormone replacement therapy. More research and clinical application are required to confirm significant effects of these medications.

PATIENT FOLLOW-UP, PROGNOSIS, AND QUALITY-OF-LIFE DECISIONS

It is important to have frequent follow-up visits and monitor treatment prognosis.

Regular checkups and laboratory examinations are important in cases with pharmacologic interventions. Clients should be informed of the prognosis and should be educated to evaluate pain, discomfort, and general quality of life of an aging pet. Depending on the severity of the problem, euthanasia may have to be considered in some cases after considering the quality of life of the pets.

SUMMARY

Compared with their younger counterparts, it is difficult to diagnose behavioral problems in older pets. This is true, in part, because the first signs of many underlying degenerative disease conditions in aging animals are reflected as a behavioral change. More frequent detailed clinical examinations are recommended for older pets and establishment of a baseline assessment is important to compare with future disease conditions related to aging.

Proper history taking, general clinical examination, laboratory examination, and consideration of CDS signs are important steps in diagnosis. A combination of client education, behavioral and environmental enrichment, balanced nutrition, and pharmacologic intervention can improve the behavioral problems and quality of life in an aging pet.

REFERENCES

1. Grimm D. Why we outlive our pets. Science 2015;350(6265):1182–5.
2. Cozzi B, Ballarin C, Mantovani R, et al. Aging and veterinary care of cats, dogs, and horses through the records of three university veterinary hospitals. Front Vet Sci 2017;4:14.
3. Epstein M, Kuehn NF, Landsberg G, et al, Senior Care Guidelines Task Force. AAHA Senior Care Guidelines for Dogs and Cats. J Am Anim Hosp Assoc 2005;41(2):81–91.
4. Landsberg G, Araujo JA. Behavior problems in geriatric pets. Vet Clin North Am Small Anim Pract 2005;35(3):675–98.
5. Mongillo P, Pitteri E, Carnier P, et al. Does the attachment system towards owners change in aged dogs? Physiol Behav 2013;120:64–9.
6. Topál J, Miklósi Á, Csányi V, et al. Attachment behavior in dogs (Canis familiaris): a new application of Ainsworth's (1969) Strange Situation Test. J Comp Psychol 1998;112(3):219.

7. Gácsi M, Topál J, Miklósi Á, et al. Attachment behavior of adult dogs (Canis familiaris) living at rescue centers: forming new bonds. J Comp Psychol 2001;115(4):423.

8. Topál J, Gácsi M, Miklósi Á, et al. Attachment to humans: a comparative study on hand-reared wolves and differently socialized dog puppies. Anim Behav 2005; 70(6):1367–75.

9. Beale BS. Orthopedic problems in geriatric dogs and cats. Vet Clin North Am Small Anim Pract 2005;35(3):655–74.

10. Lund EM, Armstrong J, Kirk C, et al. Prevalence and risk factors for obesity in adult dogs from private US veterinary practices. Int J Appl Res Vet Med 2006; 4(2):177–86.

11. Laflamme DP. Nutritional care for aging cats and dogs. Vet Clin North Am Small Anim Pract 2012;42(4):769–91.

12. Kyllar M, Witter K. Prevalence of dental disorders in pet dogs. Vet Med (Praha) 2005;50(11):496–505.

13. Holmstrom SE. Veterinary dentistry in senior canines and felines. Vet Clin North Am Small Anim Pract 2012;42(4):793–808.

14. Kass PH, Peterson ME, Levy J, et al. Evaluation of environmental, nutritional, and host factors in cats with hyperthyroidism. J Vet Intern Med 1999;13(4):323–9.

15. Boari A, Aste G. Diagnosis and management of geriatric canine endocrine disorders. Vet Res Commun 2003;27(Suppl 1):543–54.

16. Panciera DL, Thomas CB, Eicker SW, et al. Epizootiologic patterns of diabetes mellitus in cats: 333 cases (1980-1986). J Am Vet Med Assoc 1990;197(11): 1504–8.

17. Pugliese A, Gruppillo A, Di Pietro S. Clinical nutrition in gerontology: chronic renal disorders of the dog and cat. Vet Res Commun 2005;29(2):57–63.

18. Carpenter RE, Pettifer GR, Tranquilli WJ. Anesthesia for geriatric patients. Vet Clin North Am Small Anim Pract 2005;35(3):571–80.

19. Guglielmini C. Cardiovascular diseases in the ageing dog: diagnostic and therapeutic problems. Vet Res Commun 2003;27(1):555–60.

20. Hoskins JD, McCurnin DM. Geriatric care in the late 1990s. Vet Clin North Am Small Anim Pract 1997;27(6):1273–84.

21. Jonsson L. Coronary arterial lesions and myocardial infarcts in the dog; a pathologic and microangiographic study. Acta Vet Scand 1972;38:1–80.

22. Strasser A, Teltscher A, May B, et al. Age-associated changes in the immune system of German shepherd dogs. Transbound Emerg Dis 2000;47(3):181–92.

23. Mittman C, Edelman NH, Norris AH, et al. Relationship between chest wall and pulmonary compliance and age. J Appl Physiol 1965;20(6):1211–6.

24. Araujo JA, Landsberg GM, Milgram NW, et al. Improvement of short-term memory performance in aged beagles by a nutraceutical supplement containing phosphatidylserine, Ginkgo biloba, vitamin E, and pyridoxine. Can Vet J 2008;49(4): 379–85.

25. Heath SE, Barabas S, Craze PG. Nutritional supplementation in cases of canine cognitive dysfunction—a clinical trial. Appl Anim Behav Sci 2007;105(4):284–96.

26. Reme CA, Dramard V, Kern L, et al. Effect of S-adenosylmethionine tablets on the reduction of age-related mental decline in dogs: a double-blinded, placebo-controlled trial. Vet Ther 2008;9(2):69–82.

27. Milgram NW, Landsberg G, Merrick D, et al. A novel mechanism for cognitive enhancement in aged dogs with the use of a calcium buffering protein. J Vet Behav 2015;10(3):217–22.

28. Messonier S. Natural health bible for dogs and cats. Roseville (CA): Prima; 2001. p. 56–7.

29. Fox SM. Painful decisions for senior pets. Vet Clin North Am Small Anim Pract 2012;42(4):727–48.

30. Gunn-Moore DA. Cognitive dysfunction in cats: clinical assessment and management. Top Companion Anim Med 2011;26(1):17–24.

31. Salvin HE, McGreevy PD, Sachdev PS, et al. Growing old gracefully—Behavioral changes associated with "successful aging" in the dog, Canis familiaris. J Vet Behav 2011;6(6):313–20.

32. Landsberg GM, Deporter T, Araujo JA. Clinical signs and management of anxiety, sleeplessness, and cognitive dysfunction in the senior pet. Vet Clin North Am Small Anim Pract 2011;41(3):565–90.

33. Skoumalova A, Rofina J, Schwippelova Z, et al. The role of free radicals in canine counterpart of senile dementia of the Alzheimer type. Exp Gerontol 2003;38(6): 711–9.

34. Borras D, Ferrer I, Pumarola M. Age-related changes in the brain of the dog. Vet Pathol 1999;36(3):202–11.

35. Milgram NW, Head E, Weiner E, et al. Cognitive functions and aging in the dog: acquisition of nonspatial visual tasks. Behav Neurosci 1994;108(1):57–68.

36. Landsberg GM, Nichol J, Araujo JA. Cognitive dysfunction syndrome: a disease of canine and feline brain aging. Vet Clin North Am Small Anim Pract 2012;42(4): 749–68.

37. Landsberg GM, Denenberg S, Araujo JA. Cognitive dysfunction in cats: a syndrome we used to dismiss as 'old age'. J Feline Med Surg 2010;12(11): 837–48.

38. Notari L, Mills D. Possible behavioral effects of exogenous corticosteroids on dog behavior: a preliminary investigation. J Vet Behav 2011;6(6):321–7.

39. Cotman CW, Head E, Muggenburg BA, et al. Brain aging in the canine: a diet enriched in antioxidants reduces cognitive dysfunction. Neurobiol Aging 2002; 23(5):809–18.

40. Araujo JA, Baulk J, de Rivera C. The aged dog as a natural model of alzheimer's disease progression. In: Landsberg G, Mad'ari A, Žilka N, editors. Canine and feline dementia: molecular basis, diagnostics and therapy. Cham (Germany): Springer International Publishing; 2017. p. 69–93.

41. McMillan FD. Maximizing quality of life in ill animals. J Am Anim Hosp Assoc 2003;39(3):227–35.

42. Milgram NW, Head E, Zicker SC, et al. Long-term treatment with antioxidants and a program of behavioral enrichment reduces age-dependent impairment in discrimination and reversal learning in beagle dogs. Exp Gerontol 2004;39(5): 753–65.

43. Milgram NW, Zicker SC, Head E, et al. Dietary enrichment counteracts age-associated cognitive dysfunction in canines. Neurobiol Aging 2002;23(5):737–45.

44. Pan Y, Larson B, Araujo JA, et al. Dietary supplementation with medium-chain TAG has long-lasting cognition-enhancing effects in aged dogs. Br J Nutr 2010;103(12):1746–54.

45. Milgram NW, Ivy GO, Head E, et al. The effect of L-deprenyl on behavior, cognitive function, and biogenic amines in the dog. Neurochem Res 1993;18(12): 1211–9.

46. Winblad B, Fioravanti M, Dolezal T, et al. Therapeutic use of nicergoline. Clin Drug Investig 2008;28(9):533–52.

47. Carrillo MC, Ivy GO, Milgram NW, et al. (-)Deprenyl increases activities of super-oxide dismutase (SOD) in striatum of dog brain. Life Sci 1994;54(20):1483–9.

48. Landsberg G. Therapeutic options for cognitive decline in senior pets. J Am Anim Hosp Assoc 2006;42(6):407–13.

49. Denenberg S, Landsberg G. Current pharmacological and non-pharmacological approaches for therapy of feline and canine dementia. In: Landsberg G, Maďari A, Žilka N, editors. Canine and feline dementia: molecular basis, diagnostics and therapy. Cham (Germany): Springer International Publishing; 2017. p. 129–43.

50. Siwak CT, Gruet P, Woehrlé F, et al. Behavioral activating effects of adrafinil in aged canines. Pharmacol Biochem Behav 2000;66(2):293–300.

51. Siwak CT, Gruet P, Woehrle F, et al. Comparison of the effects of adrafinil, propentofylline, and nicergoline on behavior in aged dogs. Am J Vet Res 2000;61(11):1410–4.

Advances in Behavioral Psychopharmacology

Leslie Sinn, DVM

KEYWORDS

- Psychopharmacology • Behavioral drugs • Behavioral therapy
- Psychoactive medication • Canine • Feline

KEY POINTS

- Recent findings focusing on such drugs as trazodone, clonidine, and gabapentin have revolutionized how clinicians handle and treat dogs and cats.
- The results of these studies should be applied in the clinical setting with caution and with a full understanding of the potential pros and cons of using these medications.
- Despite promising results, additional research is desperately needed regarding pharmacokinetics, frequent and infrequent side effects, long-term behavioral impact, and the most clinically appropriate and effective use of these drugs.

INTRODUCTION

Research in the area of veterinary behavioral psychopharmacology is in its infancy. Only clomipramine (separation anxiety), selegiline (cognitive decline), and dexmedetomidine (noise phobia) are approved for use in dogs in the United States. There are no approved behavioral drugs for cats. Using any of the previously mentioned medications for purposes other than the indications listed on the label and the use of any psychoactive medication not listed previously is considered extralabel use and falls under the rules of the Animal Medicinal Drug Use Clarification Act of 1994 and its implementing regulations.

Extralabel use refers to the use of an approved animal or human drug in a manner that is not in accordance with the label directions and is limited to situations where the animal's health is at risk and/or suffering or death may result from lack of treatment[1]: "Actual use or intended use of a drug in an animal in a manner that is, not in accordance with the approved labeling. This includes, but is not limited to, use in species not listed in the labeling, use for indications (disease and other conditions) not listed in the labeling, use at dosage levels, frequencies, or routes of administration other than those stated in the labeling, and deviation from labeled withdrawal time based on these different uses" (21 CFR 530.3[a]). Client consent should always be obtained before proceeding with extralabel drug use.

The author has nothing to disclose.
Behavior Solutions, PO Box 116, Hamilton, VA 20159, USA
E-mail address: lsinndvm@gmail.com

Vet Clin Small Anim 48 (2018) 457–471
https://doi.org/10.1016/j.cvsm.2017.12.011

vetsmall.theclinics.com

Recent studies have led to some groundbreaking findings regarding the use of medications for the support of behavioral health. Despite tantalizing results, these studies should be viewed in light of their limitations. Behavioral studies typically involve small numbers of animals often maintained in nonstandardized condition.[2] Most are open trials or retrospective studies. Many rely on owner or veterinarian observation opening up the possibility of placebo effect, which can reach 45%.[3] Consequently, the results of these studies should be applied in the clinical setting with caution and with a full understanding of the potential pros and cons of using these medications.[4]

α_2-ADRENERGIC AGONISTS

α_2-Adrenergic agonists bind to presynaptic α_2 receptors (negative feedback receptors) in the brainstem causing a decrease in calcium levels; inhibiting the release of norepinephrine (NE); and resulting in a subsequent decrease in sympathetic tone, sedation, analgesia, and anesthesia.[5] Drugs in this class include clonidine, detomidine, and dexmedetomidine. Hypotension, cardiac depression, and atrioventricular block can occur with higher doses. Sedation, ataxia, bradycardia, and blanching at the site of oral transmucosal (OTM) administration may also occur. Species vary in the type, number, density, and distribution of α receptors so response to these medications varies.[6] One advantage of the use of α_2-adrenergic agonists is that atipamezole (Antisedan-Zoetis) is an effective reversal agent.[6]

Clonidine

Clonidine is a hypertension medication that has been used in human medicine for decades. It is a centrally acting α_2-adrenergic agonist. It is nonselective, acting on α_{2A}, α_{2B}, and α_{2C} adrenergic receptors and the imidazoline receptor.[5]

There is a single research study published on the efficacy of this medication in dogs.[7] In this study 22 dogs were divided into two groups of 11 each, one with separation anxiety, noise phobias, and storm phobias, and the second group with fear-aggression and/or fear-based territorial aggression. According to assessments made by owners, 70% of owners in the first group indicated that clonidine was more effective than previously administered medication, whereas 92% of the owners in the second group indicated that clonidine reduced the intensity of their dog's aggressive response. Previously administered medications included propranolol, alprazolam, or buspirone alone or in addition to baseline sertraline, fluoxetine, or clomipramine. Adverse side effects were limited to a single dog with noise phobia reporting increased sensitivity to noise while on the medication. Clonidine was administered 1.5 to 2 hours before the fear-inducing event. The optimal median dosage of clonidine ranged from 0.017 mg/kg to 0.026 mg/kg orally on an as-needed basis (PRN) up to twice daily. Duration of efficacy was 4 to 6 hours. Pharmacokinetics for clonidine were extrapolated from human use because data in dogs are lacking.[7] In humans, clonidine is administered two to three times daily. Drowsiness, sedation, fatigue, hypotension, bradycardia, and respiratory depression are all potential side effects but are dose dependent and were not observed in this study at these dosages.

Takeaway points

PRN use of clonidine seems to be effective in the treatment of fear-based behaviors in dogs, especially in situations where alprazolam or propranolol provided no benefit. Side effects at these dosages were not observed (increased sensitivity to noise was reported in one dog). The optimal median dosage of clonidine was 0.017 mg/kg to 0.026 mg/kg orally PRN administered 1.5 to 2 hours before the fear-inducing event up to twice daily.

Detomidine

Detomidine is an α_2-adrenergic agonist that works in a manner similar to clonidine but is more selective for the α_2 receptor subset. It is commercially available in an OTM formulation used for restraint and sedation in horses Dormosedan (Zoetis).

There are two studies looking at its efficacy in dogs. The first study evaluated its effect in six laboratory dogs given 0.35 mg/m^2 via OTM route. Five of six dogs achieved adequate sedation.[8] Four of six dogs achieved sedation within 45 minutes with a duration of approximately 30 minutes. Side effects reported included transient bradycardia in five of six dogs and second-degree atrioventricular block in one dog. No interventions were necessary in any of the dogs and all recovered without incident.

In the second study 12 healthy dogs were evaluated using a blinded crossover prospective trial. Dogs were randomly divided into OTM (0.5 mg/m^2) or intravenous (IV; 0.125 mg/m^2) groups and administered detomidine.[9] All dogs became lateral posttreatment. Duration of lateral recumbency was approximately 1.5 hours. No major adverse side effects were observed. Sedation scores for dogs receiving OTM were lower (less sedated) that those receiving IV detomidine; however, sedation scores did not vary between treatments during jugular catheterization. Five of six OTM dogs were successfully restrained in lateral recumbency and a jugular catheter placed. Maximum drug concentration and peak sedation occurred 1 hour after OTM administration. All dogs developed bradycardia but none required treatment. The OTM dogs exhibited blanching at the OTM administration site. Emesis was not observed in either treatment group.

There is one pilot study looking at the effects of OTM detomidine in seven adult cats.[10] Each cat (average weight 4.12 kg $\pm$ 0.72) received 4 mg m$^{2-1}$ of OTM detomidine gel. Moderate sedation occurred in all cats with peak plasma concentration occurring at a mean of 45 minutes. Decreased heart rate and blood pressure and increased blood glucose were observed in all cats. These effects subsided within 120 minutes. Emesis occurred in all seven cats within 2 minutes of OTM gel administration.

Takeaway points

OTM (0.5 mg/m^2) detomidine provides adequate chemical restraint for short-duration clinical procedures in healthy dogs. Likely side effects include bradycardia, increased blood pressure, increased blood glucose, and mucosal blanching at the OTM site. Although OTM detomidine seems to provide moderate sedation in cats based on a single pilot study, additional research is warranted.

Dexmedetomidine

Dexmedetomidine is the pharmacologically active dextroisomer of medetomidine and a highly selective α_2-adrenergic agonist. Dexmedetomidine induces sedation by binding to presynaptic α_2-adrenergic neurons in the locus ceruleus in the brainstem inhibiting voltage gated Ca2$^+$ channels, decreasing the firing rate of locus ceruleus neurons, and causing presynaptic inhibition.[11] The end result is a decrease in NE release centrally and peripherally.[12] Reduced level of NE leads to reduced fear and anxiety. Sedation by dexmedetomidine mirrors natural sleep.[11]

Dexmedetomidine hydrochloride oromucosal gel Sileo (Zoetis), is a newly available Food and Drug Administration (FDA)-approved medication for the treatment of canine noise phobias. It is not approved for use in cats. It comes in a 3-mL syringe (0.1 mg/mL). It is administered in the buccal cavity between the cheek and gum. OTM administration reaches peak plasma concentration within 0.6 hours with approximately 28% bioavailability, peak plasma concentration is approximately one-quarter of the same dosage with IV or intramuscular (IM) administration. A single dose lasts approximately 2 to 3 hours.[13]

In a randomized, double-blind, placebo-controlled, clinical field study 182 dogs with fireworks phobia were divided into a placebo and a treatment group.[14] Dogs received either 0.1 mg/mL dexmedetomidine OTM gel at a dose of 125 μg/m² or an equivalent volume of placebo gel applied to oral mucosa as needed up to five times. Dogs receiving treatment were assessed by 72% of owners as having an excellent to good response versus 37% of those receiving placebo. The only reported side effect was emesis in 4 of 89 dogs receiving dexmedetomidine.

In a case series, four aggressive dogs in a clinical setting were administered dexmedetomidine OTM gel at a mean dose of 32.6 μg/kg. Satisfactory sedation was achieved in all four dogs.[12] Two dogs were successfully reversed using atipamezole following completion of their medical procedures. The other two had been presented expressly for euthanasia, which was carried out during the sedation by detomidine. There were no observed adverse side effects.

In cats, three studies looked at the effects of OTM dexmedetomidine. The first study was a randomized, crossover study involving 12 cats given dexmedetomidine (40 μg/kg) either OTM or IM.[15] There were no statistical differences between groups in sedation or nociception. Time to onset of sedation in the OTM group was 30 ± 40 minutes and duration was 99 ± 124 minutes. Nine of 12 cats in the IM group and 11 of 12 cats in the OTM group vomited. One cat in the IM group displayed hypersalivation.

The second study was a randomized, blinded, prospective clinical study involving 87 female shelter-owned cats.[16] The cats were randomly allocated to two groups and administered dexmedetomidine (20 μg/kg⁻¹) + buprenorphine (20 μg/kg⁻¹) either OTM or IM. Statistically there was no significant difference in sedation between groups. Sedation was observed in both groups approximately 20 minutes after administration. The cats in the IM group were observably more sedated; however, roughly 20% of cats in both groups required additional sedation. Approximately 20% of cats vomited regardless of route of administration. The researchers indicated that hypersalivation was a common side effect in the OTM group.

The third study was a randomized, blinded crossover study, with 1 month washout between treatments involving six female spayed cats.[17] A combination of dexmedetomidine (40 μg/kg⁻¹) and buprenorphine (20 μg/kg⁻¹) was administered by either OTM or IM. There was no difference in nociception or sedation between the two groups. Peak sedation occurred 30 to 60 minutes after OTM administration. Salivation was noted in two of six cats and vomiting was reported in four of six (OTM) and three of six (IM) cats, respectively. Four hours after administration three of the cats in the IM group and all of the cats in the OTM group were able to stand.

Takeaway points

Dexmedetomidine OTM gel at a dose of 125 mg/m² given PRN up to five times per event provides excellent to good relief of anxiety associated with fear of fireworks in most cases. Emesis may be an infrequent side effect. Extralabel use of dexmedetomidine OTM gel at a mean dose of 32.6 μg/kg may be used to provide chemical restraint of aggressive dogs requiring medical procedures.

Extralabel use of dexmedetomidine OTM gel in cats at a dosage between 20 μg/kg⁻¹ and 40 μg/kg⁻¹ provides adequate sedation for clinical procedures of moderate duration. Vomiting is a common side effect.

β-ADRENERGIC RECEPTOR ANTAGONISTS

β-Adrenergic receptor antagonists (β-blockers) were developed in the 1950s for the treatment of cardiac and circulatory diseases in humans. β-blockers, such as propranolol and pindolol, have also been used in the treatment of post-traumatic stress disorder and panic disorders in people and canine post-traumatic stress disorder.[18,19]

Propranolol

Propranolol is a ß1, 2-adrenoreceptor antagonist that works centrally and peripherally to inhibit the actions of NE. In addition, propranolol has a centrally acting inhibitory effect on the protein synthesis needed to consolidate recent events into long-term memory.[19] It is being studied in humans for the treatment of phobias, such as fear of injections, dental visits, presentation phobia, and arachnophobia.[19] A recent review of the literature, however, calls into question the efficacy of propranolol in people.[19] In dogs the efficacy of propranolol is questionable because there is evidence that resting dogs do not have the inherent adrenergic tone that might be suppressed by ß-blockers.[20]

Pindolol

Pindolol, a partial ß-adrenoceptor antagonist receptor blocker with action at the presynaptic autoreceptor and with intrinsic sympathomimetic activity, could be potentially more effective than propranolol.[20] It is also a 5-HT1A receptor weak partial agonist/antagonist. In addition, inhibition of nitric oxide synthesis has an anxiolytic effect in animals and pindolol is a potent scavenger of nitric oxide.[21] There is some evidence that pindolol accelerates the response to selective serotonin reuptake inhibitors (SSRIs) in people.[22]

Takeaway points

There are no published studies on the use of these medications for behavioral purposes in dogs or cats.

ALPHA-2-DELTA LIGANDS

Gabapentin and pregabalin are known as $\alpha2\delta1$ ligands because they bind to the $\alpha2\delta1$ presynaptic voltage-sensitive calcium channels blocking release of excitatory neurotransmitters (glutamate, substance P, NE).[5] They have been used as anxiolytics for the treatment of social anxiety and panic disorder in people.[5]

Gabapentin

Gabapentin is a structural analogue of γ-aminobutyric acid but it does not alter γ-aminobutyric acid binding. Its anxiolytic effect is believed to be caused by the binding of voltage-sensitive calcium channels in the amygdala preventing the release of glutamate and the associated fear response.[5] It is available as a generic or as the human branded product, Neurontin (Pfizer). Avoid the use of the human oral solution in dogs because it contains 300 mg/mL of xylitol. Peak levels occur about 100 minutes after dosing in cats and 90 minutes in dogs.[23,24] The mean elimination half-life of 3 hours is similar in dogs and cats.[23,24] Gabapentin has been prescribed for refractory and complex partial seizures and chronic pain, especially neuropathic pain. Adverse side effects include ataxia and sedation at higher doses and the risk of seizures if the medication is abruptly stopped after chronic administration.[25]

There are two studies looking at the behavioral effects of gabapentin in cats. In a double-blind, placebo-controlled study, 53 cats in a spay/neuter program were administered either placebo or 50 or 100 mg of gabapentin orally.[26] Stress scores were reduced in both gabapentin groups. Level of sedation was no different between treatment or placebo groups. Four cats were observed to hypersalivate, two in the placebo group, one in the low-treatment group, and one in the high-treatment group.

The second study was a randomized, blinded crossover clinical study involving 20 pet cats with a history of stressful or fractious behavior during veterinary visits.[27]

Cats were given either placebo or 100 mg of gabapentin 90 minutes before being placed in a carrier and transported to the veterinary hospital. One week later, the same protocol was followed using the opposite treatment. A standardized veterinary examination was completed with veterinarians assigning a compliance score and owners assigning a stress score to the cat's behavior during the visit. Scores were lower in all categories (less stressed, better compliance) when cats received gabapentin versus placebo. Side effects (6 of 20) associated with gabapentin administration included hypersalivation (1 of 20), vomiting (2 of 20), sedation, and ataxia, all which resolved within 8 hours postadministration. A single cat was unable to be examined (1 of 20) despite gabapentin administration.

Takeaway points

Gabapentin at a dosage of 50 to 100 mg orally per cat reduces visible signs of stress 1 to 2 hours after administration. Gabapentin at a dosage of 100 mg orally per cat helped to facilitate transport and compliance during veterinary examination. There are no studies that evaluate the use of gabapentin to alter behavior in dogs.

SEROTONIN ANTAGONIST REUPTAKE INHIBITORS

Drugs that block serotonin receptors and serotonin reuptake are referred to as serotonin antagonist reuptake inhibitors. Trazodone is the most commonly used medication from this category in veterinary medicine.

Trazodone

Trazodone is an anxiolytic, antidepressant, and anticompulsive medication that was introduced in human medicine in the 1960s. It is often used to treat insomnia and is thought to work synergistically with SSRIs and tricyclic acids. It is classified as a serotonin antagonist reuptake inhibitor because of its action as an antagonist at serotonin 2A and 2C receptors and its secondary effect on the inhibition of serotonin reuptake.[5] Seven studies were found investigating the efficacy of trazodone: five in dogs and two in cats.

The first study was a retrospective case series looking at trazodone use in 56 cases of canine anxiety.[28] The dogs reviewed had multiple behavioral disorders and were distributed as follows: 14 dogs received trazodone as a daily medication, 20 received trazodone as needed for anxiety, and 22 received trazodone both daily and as needed. Concomitant medications included SSRIs, tricyclic acids, buspirone, reserpine, and melatonin. The mean daily dosage of trazodone regardless of behavioral diagnosis or PRN or maintenance use was between 7.25 and 7.6 mg/kg/d. No dog received more than 300 mg/dose. The maximum dose for any individual dog was 19.5 mg/kg/d. In three dogs trazodone was discontinued because of side effects: the first with colitis, a second with gagging, and a third with behavioral disinhibition that consisted of previously unreported counter-surfing. Three dogs did not respond to trazodone administration and were dogs that had been resistant to other medications and behavior modification.

The second study looked at the use of trazodone to facilitate postsurgical confinement in dogs.[29] This was a prospective, open-label clinical trial conducted with 36 client-owned animals. Dogs were placed on trazodone the day after surgery at a dosage of 3.5 mg/kg orally every 12 hours with tramadol 4 to 6 mg/kg orally every 8 to 12 hours. Tramadol was discontinued after 3 days and trazodone was increased to 7 mg/kg orally every 12 hours and maintained for 4 weeks. If necessary, trazodone was increased to 7 to 10 mg/kg every 8 to 12 hours. In client-completed surveys, 89% of owners reported that trazodone helped to improve tolerance of confinement in their dogs. No dogs were withdrawn from the study because of adverse side effects. Median duration of action was approximately 4 hours and median onset of action was 31 to 45 minutes.

The third study was a prospective observational study involving 120 client-owned hospitalized dogs divided equally into a treatment group and environmentally matched control animals.[30] Trazodone was administered at a dosage of 4 mg/kg every 12 hours, with the dose or frequency increased to 10 to 12 mg/kg or to every 8 hours if additional anxiolysis was needed. Observations were performed by one of two investigators approximately 45 minutes after trazodone was administered with the second observation occurring 90 minutes after the first. Treatment with trazadone had a significant effect on the reduction of some stress behaviors including lip licking, panting, whining, and cumulative frenetic and freeze behavior summation scores.

The fourth study investigated the use of trazodone in the postoperative confinement of dogs.[31] It was a placebo-controlled, double-blind clinical trial involving 29 client-owned animals evaluated by clients for a 4-week postsurgical period. Although trazodone was well tolerated, no statistical difference in behavior was found between the trazodone and placebo group. A total of 70% of owners in both groups receiving either medication or placebo indicated that the respective treatment helped to facilitate calming. Dogs received a mean dosage of 15.13 mg/kg trazodone divided twice daily.

In the fifth study in dogs, the investigators looked at the pharmacokinetics of oral and intravenously administered trazodone.[32] Trazodone was well tolerated orally at a dosage of 8 mg/kg. Time to maximum plasma concentration was 445 ± 271 minutes, and indicated significant individual variability. The only adverse effect reported after oral administration was hypersalivation in one dog. Neither cardiovascular depression nor hypotension were detected. Researchers noted subjective anxiolytic and sedating effects.

There are only two studies investigating the effect of trazodone on cats. The first is a pilot study involving six laboratory cats.[33] Single test doses of 50, 75, and 100 mg trazodone and placebo were administered. Accelerometer data for all three doses showed activity reduction (43%–86%) but no difference in the behavioral response to examination 90 minutes postadministration regardless of the dosage administered. There was a significant difference in the behavioral video observation scores in placebo versus the 100-mg dose. Latency to peak sedation for the 100-mg dose was approximately 2 hours.

The second study was a double-blind, placebo-controlled, randomized crossover study using 10 client-owned cats.[34] Each cat was given 50 mg of trazodone or a placebo and then subjected to transport in a carrier and a structured examination. Owners and veterinarians assessed the cats for anxiety and ease of handling. After a 1- to 3-week washout period, the protocol was repeated with the opposite treatment. The administration of trazodone resulted in decreased anxiety during transport and increased ease of handling ($P = .031$). The most common side effect was sleepiness.

Takeaway points

Trazodone is well tolerated in dogs at dosages ranging from 3.5 mg/kg to 12 mg/kg every 8 to 12 hours. Trazodone has been used in dogs for postoperative confinement, hospitalization, and the treatment of multiple behavioral disorders in conjunction with a variety of different medication.

Of concern is a recent double-blind, placebo-controlled study examining postoperative confinement in dogs that found no difference in behavior between the trazodone and the placebo group.[31]

Significant individual variability in metabolism of trazodone exists, therefore test doses are recommended before implementing its use.[32] The administration of trazodone at a dosage of 50 mg/cat resulted in decreased anxiety during transport and increased ease in handling.[34]

Trazodone should be used with caution in conjunction with other drugs that also affect serotonin to avoid rare, but potentially fatal serotonin syndrome.

ADDITIONAL MEDICATIONS
Maropitant

Maropitant (Cerenia-Zoetis) is a neurokinin (NK1) receptor antagonist used to treat motion sickness and vomiting in dogs and cats[35,36] It is available in tablet and injectable formulations with only the injectable approved for use in cats. Maropitant acts centrally and peripherally by inhibiting substance P, the neurotransmitter associated with vomiting. Substance P and NK1 receptors are widely distributed and are found in areas associated with the regulation of emotions including the amygdala, the periaqueductal gray, and the hypothalamus. Substance P has been linked with aggressive behavior in some mammalian species.[37] NK1 receptors and substance P are also involved in the stress response. Many dogs and cats that are anxious during car rides also exhibit signs of motion sickness, such as hypersalivation, vomiting, drooling, vocalization, lip licking, and repeated swallowing. Maropitant is a practical addition for the treatment of animals experiencing car sickness. Administration of this medication before grooming, hospital visits, or other handling or mildly invasive procedures may help reduce the stress response. It is often prescribed in conjunction with benzodiazepines. Maropitant also has analgesic properties because NK1 receptors are involved in the transmission of pain via substance P.[38,39] Peak onset is 45 minutes after injection or 1 hour after oral administration. The use of tablets in cats or the use of maropitant for purposes other than the prevention of acute vomiting or motion sickness is considered extralabel use.

Takeaway points

Maropitant is indicated for the treatment of motion sickness and other causes of nausea in dogs and cats. As a drug that blocks substance P, maropitant has the potential for many additional uses including as an adjunct medication for the treatment of pain and as a mediator of the stress response during handling and hospitalization.

Memantine

Memantine is a noncompetitive, moderate affinity, voltage-dependent N-methyl-D-aspartate receptor antagonist that reduces glutamatergic neurotransmission.[40] It is used for the treatment of cognitive decline and obsessive compulsive disorders in people. Its neuroprotective aspects are believed to be caused by the prevention of calcium influx into cells caused by chronic stimulation of N-methyl-D-aspartate receptors. In addition to its antiglutamatergic action it also acts as an agonist at the dopamine D_2 receptor and as a noncompetitive antagonist at serotonin 5-HT3 and nicotinic acetylcholine receptors.[40]

In a case series of 11 dogs, either memantine alone or memantine added to ongoing fluoxetine treatment was used to treat canine compulsive disorders (CCD), which consisted of light/shadow chasing, spinning, or tail chasing.[41] Memantine was administered at a dosage of 0.3 mg/kg to 1 mg/kg orally twice daily. Based on owner assessment, 7 of 11 dogs showed a reduction in signs of CCD. The only reported side effect was increased urination in 1 of 11 dogs.

In a single case study memantine was administered to treat spinning in a dog in conjunction with fluoxetine at a dosage of 0.4 mg/kg orally twice daily. The owner reported between 50% and 75% improvement in the signs of CCD.[42]

Takeaway points
Memantine administered at a dosage of 0.3 to 1.0 mg/kg orally twice a day either alone or in conjunction with fluoxetine may help in the treatment of CCD.

Venlafaxine

Venlafaxine was one the first serotonin NE reuptake inhibitors developed (SNRIs) in the 1990s. It is approved for the treatment of depression, general anxiety, and panic disorder in humans. SNRIs have also been used in the treatment of urinary incontinence in women.[43] The half-life of venlafaxine in dogs is only 2 to 4 hours making its use likely impractical.[44] When administered IV in cats, venlafaxine caused a dose-dependent decrease in neuronal firing rate that lasted greater than 24 hours.[45] There are no data currently available on oral pharmacokinetics in cats. However, even in cases of ingestion of doses 17.4 ± 12.5 mg/kg, 6 of 12 cats were asymptomatic and 6 of 12 recovered uneventfully with symptomatic treatment.[46]

In a retrospective case series of 13 cats treated with venlafaxine for periuria 11 of 13 cats responded and 4 of 11 subsequently relapsed.[47] Six cats were treated successfully with venlafaxine for a mean duration of 20 months on dosages of 0.9 to 1.9 mg/kg orally once daily. Reported side effects were appetite suppression, increased anxiety, sedation, and increased affiliative behavior. Sixty-two percent of treated cats showed remission of clinical signs within 1 week.

Takeaway points
Venlafaxine administered orally at a dosage of 0.9 to 1.9 mg/kg once daily may be an additional option for cats with idiopathic cystitis that fail to respond to standard drug therapy.

ON THE HORIZON
Cannabis (Cannabis Sativa)

Cannabis has been used by humans for centuries with historical evidence of cultivation for medicinal purposes in China and India occurring before 1000 BC. Cannabis was introduced to the western world in the 1800s. Δ9-tetrahydrocannabinol (THC), the psychoactive substance found in cannabis, was first described in the 1960s. Identification of its binding site, the cannabinoid receptor (CB1R), did not occur until 1990.[40] Anandamide was eventually identified as the endogenous ligand of the CB1R. Several years later, a second cannabinoid, 2-arachidonoylglycerol, was also identified. Anandamide and 2-arachidonoylglycerol are referred to as endocannabinoids. Both are found in the brain and peripherally. They are produced in response to stress and primarily act to inhibit neurotransmitter release. CBR1s are not uniformly distributed in the brain with high densities of receptors found in the basal ganglia, frontal cortex, hippocampus, and cerebellum. They are also found in the interneurons of the dorsal horns of the spinal cord. More recently, a second receptor has been identified, CBR2. These receptors are found primarily peripherally in association with the immune system. Cannabis contains more than 400 different chemicals but the two of primary interest are THC and cannabidiol (CBD).[48] THC is psychoactive and binds to CBR1 and CBR2. CBD is psychoactive but has less than 10 times the potency of THC. It binds to CBR1 and CBR2 slowing endocannabinoid breakdown. In human medicine cannabinoids have been used in the treatment of anorexia; weight loss; pain; nausea; immune-mediated diseases, such as multiple sclerosis; seizures; and inflammation.[49] Information on the use of cannabinoids in dogs and cats is lacking and its medical use remains controversial. CBD has poor oral bioavailability in dogs reaching only 13% to 19%.[50] In addition it inhibits cytochrome P-450 in rats and in humans impacting the metabolism of many drugs. As a marijuana product it is still considered a Schedule 1 substance by the Federal government. In addition, these products are not approved by the FDA for the treatment or prevention of any disease in dogs or cats and have been found when tested to not contain the stated concentration of CBD or to be cross-contaminated with THC. Multiple warning letter have been issued by the FDA to manufacturers of these products.[51]

Takeaway points
The use of CBD for behavioral therapy in dogs and cats is not supported by the currently available research.

Oxytocin

Oxytocin (OT) is a neuropeptide synthetized by the hypothalamus that regulates many complex forms of social behavior and cognition in humans and animals. Increases in OT in dogs and humans have been observed in dog-human interactions and may be higher in more strongly bonded dyads.[52] Enhanced or specific OT receptor polymorphisms in the brain of the domestic dog may explain the difference between the ability of dogs to complete gazing or object choice tasks at a rate greater than chance when compared with wolves.[53]

Intranasal OT administration in humans increases trust, increases gazing time, improves social memory, and enhances the understanding of social cues.[54] Similar effects have been detected in dogs.[55–58] Intranasal OT seems to reach the central nervous system within 5 minutes of administration with plasma levels of OT being significantly elevated within 15 minutes postadministration. By 90 minutes postadministration, plasma levels of OT were no longer statistically significant.[58] The duration of effect in dogs is not known. In people, OT is administered 30 to 60 minutes before the expected stimuli or every 12 hours.[59] In the Romero studies, 40 IU of OT was administered immediately before the testing window of 60 minutes.[57,58] It is possible that the use of OT would be beneficial in a clinical setting.[60] However, the effect of OT is influenced by a host of factors including gender, genetics, and chronicity of administration.[61] Theses influences and their impact have yet to be investigated in dogs or cats.

Takeaway points
Too many questions exist regarding the effects and efficacy of OT in dogs and cats to be able to advocate for its use in clinical practice at this time.

ADDITIONAL POINTS TO KEEP IN MIND
Transdermal Absorption and Compounding

Medicating dogs and cats is challenging. Veterinarians often resort to alternative methods of medication delivery to facilitate consumption. Unfortunately, research to date indicates that compounding adversely affects drug availability. Two research studies specifically examined the delivery of fluoxetine transdermally in cats.[62,63] Both studies found reduced bioavailability with transdermal absorption versus oral administration. In one study, bioavailability transdermally was found to be 10% of oral administration.[62] Skin irritation occurred at the application site at the higher transdermal dose (10 mg/kg). In the second study, the baseline concentration of fluoxetine was found to be substantially lower with transdermal application and six of eight cats exhibited signs of irritation at the application site. It is not known if the baseline concentration achieved was sufficient to be clinically effective.[63]

Other studies have looked at the effect of compounding on a variety of drugs.[64] Most have found major discrepancies between stated concentration of medication and actual available concentration. Some formulations seem to be more stable than others (oil based) and most degrade rapidly over time. Because of the instability of compounded and alternative formulations, they should only be used as a last resort.

In addition, the simple act of halving or quartering a pill can cause substantial variation in content uniformity and stability.[65] Consequently clients should be advised to quarter or halve only one pill at a time to increase stability and decrease variability as much as feasible.

Serotonin Syndrome

Serotonin syndrome is a constellation of physiologic effects caused by an excess of serotonin.[66] Serotonin syndrome can be caused by the administration of medication at therapeutic dosages (adverse effect), the combined effect of multiple drugs (drug interaction), or the ingestion of a medication in excess (toxic effect). The effects of serotonin manifest themselves primarily on the respiratory, cardiovascular, nervous, gastrointestinal, and metabolic/endocrine systems. Primary signs include tachypnea, tachycardia, hyperexcitability, hypervigilance, agitation, aggression, muscle tremors, muscle rigidity, seizures, coma, hypersalivation, vomiting, diarrhea, and hyperthermia. In veterinary medicine most cases of serotonin syndrome are caused by accidental ingestion of an owner's medication causing a toxic effect. However, as the use of psychoactive medications becomes more prevalent in dogs and cats, the likelihood of drug interactions or adverse effects becomes more likely.[46,67] Medications that affect serotonin levels and have been implicated in cases of serotonin syndrome include SSRIs; SNRIs; atypical antipsychotics; tricyclic antidepressants; monoamine oxidase inhibitors; and miscellaneous agents, such as herbal supplements, mirtazapine, and tramadol.[66] Treatment includes decontamination if detected within 30 to 60 minutes postingestion, observation, and supportive care. If serotonin syndrome develops, cyproheptadine, a serotonin antagonist antihistamine, can be administered at a dosage of 1.1 mg/kg orally every 4 to 6 hours in dogs or 2 to 4 mg orally total dose per cat every 4 to 6 hours until symptoms have resolved.[68]

SUMMARY

Recent findings focusing on such drugs as trazodone, clonidine, and gabapentin have revolutionized how clinicians handle and treat dogs and cats. Despite promising results, additional research is desperately needed regarding pharmacokinetics, frequent and infrequent side effects, long-term impact, and the most appropriate and effective use of these drugs in the behavioral treatment and management of dogs and cats in clinical practice.[69]

REFERENCES

1. U.S. Food and Drug Administration. Animal Medicinal Drug Use Clarification Act of 1994 (AMDUCA). Anim Med Drug Use Clarification Act 1994. Available at: https://www.fda.gov/AnimalVeterinary/GuidanceComplianceEnforcement/ActsRulesRegulations/ucm085377.htm Accessed October 16, 2017.
2. Button KS, Ioannidis JPA, Mokrysz C, et al. Power failure: why small sample size undermines the reliability of neuroscience. Nat Rev Neurosci 2013;14(5):365–76.
3. Conzemius MG, Evans RB. Caregiver placebo effect for dogs with lameness from osteoarthritis. J Am Vet Med Assoc 2012;241(10):1314–9.
4. Larson RL, White BJ. The importance of the role of scientific literature in clinical decision making. J Am Vet Med Assoc 2015;247(1):58–64.

5. Stahl SM. Stahl's essential psychopharmacology: neuroscientific basis and practical applications. 4th edition. Cambridge: Cambridge University Press; 2013.

6. Dugdale A. Veterinary anaesthesia: principles to practice. 1st edition. Ames (IA): Blackwell Publishing; 2011.

7. Ogata N, Dodman NH. The use of clonidine in the treatment of fear-based behavior problems in dogs: an open trial. J Vet Behav Clin Appl Res 2011;6(2):130–7.

8. Hopfensperger MJ, Messenger KM, Papich MG, et al. The use of oral transmucosal detomidine hydrochloride gel to facilitate handling in dogs. J Vet Behav Clin Appl Res 2013;8(3):114–23.

9. Messenger KM, Hopfensperger M, Knych HK, et al. Pharmacokinetics of detomidine following intravenous or oral-transmucosal administration and sedative effects of the oral-transmucosal treatment in dogs. Am J Vet Res 2016;77(4): 413–20.

10. Smith P, Messenger K, Gould E, et al. Pharmacokinetics, sedation, and hemodynamic changes following administration of oral transmucosal detomidine gel in cats. Vet Anaesth Analg 2017;44(1):195.e5-e6.

11. Nelson LE, Lu J, Guo T, et al. The alpha2-adrenoceptor agonist dexmedetomidine converges on an endogenous sleep-promoting pathway to exert its sedative effects. Anesthesiology 2003;98(2):428–36.

12. Cohen AE, Bennett SL. Oral transmucosal administration of dexmedetomidine for sedation in 4 dogs. Can Vet J 2013;54(January):397–400.

13. U.S. Food and Drug Administration. Freedom of information summary original new animal drug application nada 141–456 SILEO (dexmedetomidine oromucosal gel) Dogs For the treatment of noise aversion in dogs. Green B Reports. 2015. Available at: https://www.fda.gov/downloads/AnimalVeterinary/Products/ApprovedAnimalDrug Products/FOIADrugSummaries/UCM475135.pdf. Accessed October 26, 2017.

14. Korpivaara M, Laapas K, Huhtinen M, et al. Dexmedetomidine oromucosal gel for noise-associated acute anxiety and fear in dogs: a randomised, double-blind, placebo-controlled clinical study. Vet Rec 2017;180(14):356.

15. Slingsby LS, Taylor PM, Monroe T. Thermal antinociception after dexmedetomidine administration in cats: a comparison between intramuscular and oral transmucosal administration. J Feline Med Surg 2009;11(10):829–34.

16. Santos LCP, Ludders JW, Erb HN, et al. Sedative and cardiorespiratory effects of dexmedetomidine and buprenorphine administered to cats via oral transmucosal or intramuscular routes. Vet Anaesth Analg 2010;37(5):417–24.

17. Porters N, Bosmans T, Debille M, et al. Sedative and antinociceptive effects of dexmedetomidine and buprenorphine after oral transmucosal or intramuscular administration in cats. Vet Anaesth Analg 2014;41(1):90–6.

18. Burghardt W. Preliminary evaluation of case series of military working dogs affected with canine post-traumatic stress disorder (N=14). In: ACVB, editor. Veterinary behavior symposium. Chicago: ACVB; 2013. p. 5–9.

19. Steenen SA, van Wijk AJ, van der Heijden GJ, et al. Propranolol for the treatment of anxiety disorders: systematic review and meta-analysis. J Psychopharmacol 2016;30(2):128–39.

20. Kantelip JP, Eschalier A. Comparison of the effects of propranolol, pindolol, oxprenolol and acebitolol on atrioventricular conduction in unanaesthetized dogs. Br J Clin Pharmacol 1982;13:159S–66S.

21. Fernandes E, Gomes A, Costa D, et al. Pindolol is a potent scavenger of reactive nitrogen species. Life Sci 2005;77(16):1983–92.

22. Isaac MT. Review: combining pindolol with an SSRI improves early outcomes in people with depression. Evid Based Ment Health 2004;7(4):107.

23. Siao KT, Pypendop BH, Ilkiw JE. Pharmacokinetics of gabapentin in cats. Am J Vet Res 2010;71(7):817–21.
24. KuKanich B, Cohen RL. Pharmacokinetics of oral gabapentin in greyhound dogs. Vet J 2011;187(1):133–5.
25. KuKanich B. Outpatient oral analgesics in dogs and cats beyond nonsteroidal antiinflammatory drugs. An evidence-based approach. Vet Clin North Am Small Anim Pract 2013;43(5):1109–25.
26. Pankratz KE, Ferris KK, Griffith EH, et al. Use of single-dose oral gabapentin to attenuate fear responses in cage-trap confined community cats: a double-blind, placebo-controlled field trial. J Feline Med Surg 2017. https://doi.org/10.1177/1098612X17719399.
27. van Haaften KA, Eichstadt LR, Stelow EA, et al. Effects of a single preappointment dose of gabapentin on signs of stress in cats during transportation and veterinary examination. J Am Vet Med Assoc 2017;251(10):1175–81.
28. Gruen ME, Sherman BL. Use of trazodone as an adjunctive agent in the treatment of canine anxiety disorders: 56 cases (1995-2007). J Am Vet Med Assoc 2008; 233(12):1902–7.
29. Gruen ME, Roe S, Griffith E, et al. Use of trazodone to facilitate postsurgical confinement in dogs. J Am Vet Med Assoc 2014;245(3):296–301.
30. Gilbert-Gregory SE, Stull JW, Rose M, et al. Effects of trazodone on behavioral signs of stress in hospitalized dogs. J Am Vet Med Assoc 2016;249(11):1281–91.
31. Gruen ME, Roe SC, Griffith E, et al. The use of trazodone to facilitate calm behavior following elective orthopedic surgery in dogs: results and lessons learned from a clinical trial. J Vet Behav Clin Appl Res 2017. https://doi.org/10.1016/j.jveb.2017.09.008.
32. Jay AR, Krotscheck U, Parsley E, et al. Pharmacokinetics, bioavailability, and hemodynamic effects of trazodone after intravenous and oral administration of a single dose to dogs. Am J Vet Res 2013;74(11):1450–6.
33. Orlando JM, Case BC, Thomson AE, et al. Use of oral trazodone for sedation in cats: a pilot study. J Feline Med Surg 2016;18(6):476–82.
34. Stevens B, Frantz ES, Orlando JM, et al. Efficacy of a single dose of trazodone hydrochloride given to cats prior to veterinary visits to reduce signs of transport-and examination-related anxiety. J Am Vet Med Assoc 2016;249(2):202–7.
35. Hickman MA, Cox SR, Mahabir S, et al. Safety, pharmacokinetics and use of the novel NK-1 receptor antagonist maropitant (Cerenia) for the prevention of emesis and motions sickness in cats. J Vet Pharmacol Ther 2008;31:220–9.
36. Ramsey DS, Kincaid K, Watkins JA, et al. Safety and efficacy of injectable and oral maropitant, a selective neurokinin1 receptor antagonist, in a randomized clinical trial for treatment of vomiting in dogs. J Vet Pharmacol Ther 2008;31(6):538–43.
37. Katsouni E. The involvement of substance P in the induction of aggressive behavior. Peptides 2009;30(8):1586–91.
38. Marquez M. Comparison of NK-1 receptor antagonist (Maropitant) to morphine as a pre-anaesthetic agent for canine ovariohysterectomy. PLoS One 2015;10(10): e0140734.
39. Niyom S, Boscan P, Twedt DC, et al. Effect of maropitant, a neurokinin-1 receptor antagonist, on the minimum alveolar concentration of sevoflurane during stimulation of the ovarian ligament in cats. Vet Anaesth Analg 2013;40(4):425–31.
40. Stolerman IP, Price LH, editors. Encyclopedia of psychopharmacology. Berlin: Springer; 2015.
41. Schneider BM, Dodman NH, Maranda L. Use of memantine in treatment of canine compulsive disorders. J Vet Behav Clin Appl Res 2009;4(3):118–26.

42. Maurer BM, Dodman NH. Animal behavior case of the month. J Am Vet Med Assoc 2007;231(4):4–7.

43. Nitti V. Duloxetine: a new pharmacologic therapy for stress urinary incontinence. Rev Urol 2004;6:S48–55.

44. Howell SR. Metabolic disposition of 14C-venlafaxine in mouse, rat, dog, rhesus monkey and man. Xenobiotica 1993;23(4):349–59.

45. Bjorvatn B, Fornal CA, Martín FJ, et al. Venlafaxine and its interaction with WAY 100635: effects on serotonergic unit activity and behavior in cats. Eur J Pharmacol 2000;404(1–2):121–32.

46. Pugh CM, Sweeney JT, Bloch CP, et al. Selective serotonin reuptake inhibitor (SSRI) toxicosis in cats: 33 cases (2004-2010). J Vet Emerg Crit Care (San Antonio) 2013;23(5):565–70.

47. Hopfensperger MJ. Use of oral venlafaxine in cats with feline idiopathic cystitis or behavioral causes of periuria. In: ACVB, editor. Veterinary behavior symposium. San Antonio (TX): ACVB; 2016. p. 13–7.

48. National Academies of Sciences, Engineering, and Medicine. The health effects of cannabis and cannabinoids: the current state of evidence and recommendations for research. Washington, DC: National Academies Press; 2017.

49. Fitzgerald KT, Bronstein AC, Newquist KL. Marijuana poisoning. Top Companion Anim Med 2013;28(1):8–12.

50. Samara E, Bialer M, Mechoulam R. Pharmacokinetics of cannabidiol in dogs. Drug Metab Dispos 1988;16(3):469–72.

51. U.S. Food And Drug Administration. Warning letters and test results for cannabidiol-related products. Public Heal Focus. 2017. Available at: https://www.fda.gov/NewsEvents/PublicHealthFocus/ucm484109.htm. Accessed October 27, 2017.

52. Odendaal JSJ, Meintjes RA. Neurophysiological correlates of affiliative behaviour between humans and dogs. Vet J 2003;165(3):296–301.

53. Kis A, Bence M, Lakatos G, et al. Oxytocin receptor gene polymorphisms are associated with human directed social behavior in dogs (Canis familiaris). PLoS One 2014;9(1):e83993.

54. Kis A, Ciobica A, Topál J. The effect of oxytocin on human-directed social behaviour in dogs (Canis Familiaris). Horm Behav 2017;94:40–52.

55. Hernádi A. Intranasally administered oxytocin affects how dogs (Canis familiaris) react to the threatening approach of their owner and an unfamiliar experimenter. Behav Process 2015;119:1–5.

56. Nagasawa M, Mitsui S, En S, et al. Oxytocin-gaze positive loop and the coevolution of human-dog bonds. Science 2015;348(6232):333–6.

57. Romero T. Oxytocin promotes social bonding in dogs. Proc Natl Acad Sci U S A 2014;111(25):9085–90.

58. Romero T, Nagasawa M, Mogi K, et al. Intranasal administration of oxytocin promotes social play in domestic dogs. Commun Integr Biol 2015;8(3):e1017157.

59. MacDonald K, MacDonald TM. The peptide that binds: a systematic review of oxytocin and its prosocial effects in humans. Harv Rev Psychiatry 2010;18(1):1–21.

60. Thielke LE, Udell MAR. The role of oxytocin in relationships between dogs and humans and potential applications for the treatment of separation anxiety in dogs. Biol Rev Camb Philos Soc 2017;92(1):378–88.

61. Bales KL. Chronic intranasal oxytocin causes long-term impairments in partner preference formation in male prairie voles. Biol Psychiatry 2013;74(3):180–8.

62. Ciribassi J, Luescher A, Pasloske KS, et al. Comparative bioavailability of fluoxetine after transdermal and oral administration to healthy cats. Am J Vet Res 2003;64(8):994–8. Available at: http://www.ncbi.nlm.nih.gov/pubmed/12926591.

63. Cats C, Eichstadt LR, Corriveau LA, et al. Absorption of transdermal fluoxetine compounded in a lipoderm base compared to oral fluoxetine in client-owned cats. Int J Pharm Compd 2017;21(3):242–6.

64. KuKanich K, KuKanich B, Slead T, et al. Evaluation of drug content (potency) for compounded and FDA-approved formulations of doxycycline on receipt and after 21 days of storage. J Am Vet Med Assoc 2017;251(7):835–42.

65. Margiocco ML, Warren J, Borgarelli M, et al. Analysis of weight uniformity, content uniformity and 30-day stability in halves and quarters of routinely prescribed cardiovascular medications. J Vet Cardiol 2009;11(1):31–9.

66. Almgreen C, Lee J. Serotonin syndrome. Clin Br 2013;11–6.

67. Thomas DE, Lee JA, Hovda LR. Retrospective evaluation of toxicosis from selective serotonin reuptake inhibitor antidepressants: 313 dogs (2005-2010). J Vet Emerg Crit Care 2012;22(6):674–81.

68. Fitzgerald KT, Bronstein AC. Selective serotonin reuptake inhibitor exposure. Top Companion Anim Med 2013;28(1):13–7.

69. Prasad V, Vandross A, Toomey C, et al. A decade of reversal: an analysis of 146 contradicted medical practices. Mayo Clin Proc 2013;88(8):790–8.

Behavioral Nutraceuticals and Diets

Jillian M. Orlando, DVM*

KEYWORDS

- Behavior • Supplement • Nutrition • Treatment • Nutraceutical • Diet • Anxiety
- Cognitive dysfunction syndrome

KEY POINTS

- Nutraceuticals are regulated as food products, not drugs, despite their ability to modify an animal's health beyond meeting nutritional needs.
- Before prescribing a nutraceutical or therapeutic diet, veterinarians should review the literature supporting the use of the product and gather information on the functional ingredients, their mechanisms of action, efficacy, and safety.
- As with psychopharmacologic agents, behavioral nutraceuticals and therapeutic diets should only be prescribed in conjunction with behavior modification and environmental management plans.
- Some nutraceuticals and diets can be prescribed in combination with psychopharmacologic agents, but attention must be paid to the product's functional ingredients and mechanism of action so that adverse interactions are avoided.

INTRODUCTION
Terminology and Regulation of Nutraceuticals and Therapeutic Diets

The term "nutraceutical" has no legal or regulatory meaning. It was coined in 1989 by a physician who combined the words "nutrition" and "pharmaceutical" for the purpose of labeling the products that seem to fall between the categories of food and drug.[1] The Dietary Supplement Health and Education Act of 1994 defined the term "dietary supplement" as a product intended to supplement the diet that contains 1 or more of the following dietary ingredients: a vitamin, mineral, herb or other botanic, amino acid, dietary substance used by man to supplement the diet by increasing the total daily intake, or a concentrate, metabolite, constituent, extract, or combination of these ingredients [21 USC 321(ff)(1)].[2] However, in 1996 the Center for Veterinary Medicine, a subset of the US Food and Drug Administration (FDA), declared this term to be inapplicable to animal products because the Dietary Supplement Health and Education

Disclosure Statement: The author has no conflicts of interest to declare.
Carolina Veterinary Behavior Clinic, Raleigh, NC, USA
* PO Box 40818, Raleigh, NC 27629.
E-mail address: jillorlandodvm@gmail.com

Act was only intended to apply to humans. Furthermore, the Center for Veterinary Medicine objects to the use of the term dietary supplement when describing animal products because it may falsely imply applicability of the Dietary Supplement Health and Education Act and its regulations of human supplements.[3] The North American Veterinary Nutraceutical Council, which was formed in 1996 and has since disbanded, defined nutraceutical as a nondrug substance that is produced in a purified or extracted form and administered orally to provide agents required for normal body structure and function with the intent of improving the health and well-being of animals.[4] Despite this fitting definition, the term nutraceutical still has no legal meaning for the purposes of regulation.

So what do we call these products and how are they categorized? Veterinarians still generally refer to these products as nutraceuticals because this seems to be the best descriptive term. However, for a legal classification, we must look back to the Federal Food Drug and Cosmetic Act of 1938. It vaguely defines "food" as articles used for food or drink for man or other animal [21 USC 321(f)].[2] A legal ruling in 1983 established a more detailed definition for food as an item consumed primarily for taste, aroma, or nutritive value.[3] Legally, nutraceuticals are regarded as food and, therefore, are not required to provide premarket safety and efficacy data to obtain clearance from the FDA as do pharmaceutical products. However, nutraceutical ingredients must have already been determined to be generally regarded as safe as defined by the FDA, be an FDA-approved food additive, or fit the definition of ingredient as listed in the Association of American Feed Control Officials book.[1] If the ingredients do not follow these rules, the product will be considered "adulterated" and, as such, is subject to FDA enforcement actions.[3] If a nutraceutical manufacturer makes claims that their product can treat or prevent a disease, then it fits the definition of a drug rather than a food. The term "drug" is defined by the Federal Food Drug and Cosmetic Act as any article intended for use in the diagnosis, cure, mitigation, treatment, or prevention of disease in man or other animal [21 USC 321(g)(1)].[2]

Legal oversight of nutraceutical products is generally lax. Enforcement of laws against nutraceuticals making drug claims are considered to be of low regulatory priority, and violations are not commonly acted on by the FDA.[3] In addition to the FDA, there are also state-level agencies, such as the state department of agriculture, that will monitor nutraceuticals. Many states follow regulations published by AAFCO and require that manufacturers register or obtain a license with their state before distributing their product.[3] Responsibility lies with the manufacturer to ensure the product is labeled appropriately. The state can review the label and, if it is found to be noncompliant, the manufacturer may be denied registration or licensure. However, the thoroughness of the review can vary. Some violations may be overlooked to maintain uniform enforcement or because they are of low priority.[3]

Nutraceutical manufactures may opt to join trade organizations such as the National Animal Supplement Council. The National Animal Supplement Council requires certain labeling and manufacturing standards of its members and has an adverse event reporting system. Manufactures who comply with regulations are allowed to use the National Animal Supplement Council seal on their product label. Nutraceutical manufacturers may also enlist the services of independent quality assurance companies such as ConsumerLab, NSF International, or the United States Pharmacopeia. These companies offer services such as facility inspections and laboratory testing to ensure ingredient strength matches label claims and to check for contamination. Qualifying products can use the company's seal on their labels.

Another area of terminology that can confuse veterinarians is that of therapeutic diets. These are the foods produced by manufacturers to provide specialized support to animals with certain medical conditions. Some veterinarians may refer to these as prescription diets because they are typically only available through a veterinarian or through online retailers that require a prescription from a veterinarian. However, this is a misnomer. "Prescription diet" is actually a registered trademark of Hill's Pet Nutrition, Inc. (Topeka, KS) and is used for their line of therapeutic diets. The names "Veterinary Diet" and "Veterinary Diets" are used by Royal Canin, USA (St. Charles, MO) and Nestle Purina PetCare Company (St. Louis, MO), respectively. The term "therapeutic diet" will be used in this article to refer to the specialty diets manufactured by various companies.

The Emergence of Nutraceuticals and Therapeutic Diets in Behavior

Behavioral problems of companion animals are becoming more widely recognized in veterinary medicine. As veterinarians begin to diagnose behavioral conditions more frequently, they look for reliable treatment options to offer their patients. There are many medications effectively used for the treatment of canine and feline behavioral conditions. However, the use of most drugs are considered to be off-label. Currently, there are only 3 proprietary products approved by the FDA for treatment of behavioral conditions: selegiline (Anipryl, Zoetis, Parsippany, NJ) for canine cognitive dysfunction, clomipramine (Clomicalm, Elanco, Greenfield, IN) for canine separation anxiety, and dexmedetomidine (Sileo, Zoetis) for canine noise aversion. The veterinary formulation of fluoxetine (packaged as the proprietary product Reconcile), used for the treatment of canine separation anxiety, is no longer manufactured. Dexmedetomidine is the only one of these medications to be approved by the FDA in the last 10 years. Obtaining FDA approval for a new medication is a long, extensive, and costly process.[1,3] New nutraceutical products, however, are not required to complete the same rigorous approval process.[3] As a result, it is much easier for a nutraceutical product to enter the market. Many nonprescription nutraceuticals and therapeutic diets intended to aid the treatment of behavioral conditions, particularly for anxiety and cognitive dysfunction syndrome, have emerged in recent years. Veterinarians are exposed to a deluge of promotional materials from manufacturers, but steps must be taken to ensure they are choosing an appropriate product for their patient. This choice should be based on an understanding of available scientific evidence regarding efficacy and safety, the product's functional ingredients and their mechanisms of action, as well as patient characteristics and client needs.

Critical Evaluation of Scientific Evidence

When trying to assess the relevance of evidence used to support the efficacy of a nutraceutical or therapeutic diet, veterinarians can start by looking at promotional materials to find the scientific research cited by the manufacturer. Veterinarians should ask themselves questions to help determine how relevant each piece of research is. Factors to question include (but are not limited to) the following:

- Species used in the study. Although many species may respond similarly to certain ingredients, there are also variations among species that can affect bioavailability, metabolism, clearance, and so on. Were the studies listed by the manufacturer performed on the same species for which the product is intended?
- Laboratory models versus clinical trials. Laboratory models of behavior can allow for standardized testing and strong scientific data. But does a laboratory animal's behavior in a manufactured setting mimic how a privately owned pet will react in a home setting?
- Testing of an ingredient versus finished product. Many products list previous experiments of single ingredients as contributing evidence of a product's efficacy.

However, some nutraceuticals contain multiple ingredients that could potentially have a synergistic effect or impact bioavailability. Does a test of a single ingredient accurately reflect how the finished product will perform? If a single ingredient was tested, was the tested dose the same as the dose in the finished product?

- Target behavioral condition. Sometimes it is necessary to narrow the scope of an investigation down to a single behavioral condition (eg, separation anxiety as opposed to all forms of anxiety). If a paper claims a product to be effective in the treatment of separation anxiety, will it be effective in the treatment of generalized anxiety or of aggression? Do the parameters tested in the experiment accurately reflect the behavioral condition (eg, does an increase in activity or heart rate reflect an increase in anxiety)?
- Mechanism of action. Different behavioral conditions are believed to have similar physiologic causes (eg, decreased serotonin levels). But do we know the physiologic changes underlying the behavior in question and do we know the mechanism of action of the product's key ingredient?
- Safety data. As with any drug, certain active ingredients can cause adverse reactions or be contraindicated with certain medical conditions or concurrent medications. Does the product list any potential side effects? What evidence is provided to assure the product is safe?
- Source of the scientific data. Cited references for a product's claims may be from peer-reviewed scientific journals, scientific meeting proceedings, or internal documents on file with the manufacturer. Does the source change how much credence to give the evidence? Should proceedings from scientific meetings or unpublished data performed by reputable scientists be considered any less valuable than an article from a widely distributed scientific journal? What if the research was performed or funded by the manufacturer? Should that consideration affect how we view the results of a study?

The purpose of these questions and of judicious review is not to discredit a manufacturer's credibility or a product's efficacy or a researcher's scientific vigor. They serve to demonstrate how important it is for veterinarians to critically evaluate the data used to support nutraceuticals or therapeutic diets. A certain amount of constructive skepticism is important and is owed to our patients.

Although veterinarians recognize the need for evidence-based medicine, not all scientific evidence is equal in strength. When looking at the scientific articles testing specific nutraceuticals or therapeutic diets, veterinarians must be able to assess the quality of research. Certain study designs and characteristics are generally regarded as boosting an experiment's strength. Such characteristics include prospective design, blinded investigators, placebo controls, balanced randomized study groups, and a large population of test subjects. The Oxford Centre for Evidence-Based Medicine has developed a scoring system that can be used to rate the power of scientific research studies. To briefly summarize the system, the highest value is awarded to systematic reviews of multiple randomized, controlled trials; followed by high-quality individual randomized, controlled trials; cohort studies; low-quality randomized, controlled trials; case series; individual case reports; and expert opinion without critical appraisal.[5] Of course, veterinarians would love to have multiple randomized, double-blinded, placebo-controlled studies with hundreds of test subjects for each and every product available. Unfortunately, large, powerful studies such as these are not always feasible in veterinary medicine. Lower societal priority compared with human medicine and a lack of funding contribute to this dilemma.[6] Therefore, we must rely on what scientific data are available to us. Not every experiment can be the gold standard. That being said, veterinarians also need to be able to critically evaluate research articles and acknowledge each paper's strengths and weaknesses.

FUNCTIONAL INGREDIENTS

The Association of American Feed Control Officials guidelines require pet foods to contain minimum levels of certain ingredients to meet an animal's physiologic needs. However, animals may show a response to nutrient supplementation in excess of the minimum requirements and the absence of a dietary deficiency.[7,8] The most commonly used functional ingredients in behavioral nutraceuticals and therapeutic diets are summarized herein. **Table 1** lists the ingredients and the products containing them. **Tables 2** and **3** list the products and their associated research.[9–37]

Alpha-Casozepine

Alpha-casozepine is a bovine milk protein derivative with a decapeptide structure created by tryptic hydrolysis of the alpha-S1 casein protein.[26] The structure is similar to that of gamma-aminobutyric acid (GABA), an inhibitory neurotransmitter that decreases signal transduction after binding to receptors. Thus, alpha-casozepine is able to bind $GABA_A$ receptors and have an inhibitory effect. This mechanism of action is similar to that of benzodiazepines, which are known to reduce anxiety.[38] However, alpha-casozepine does not create the sedative-like side effects associated with benzodiazepines.[39]

Alpha-casozepine has been tested in laboratory rats and was found to be as effective as diazepam for reducing anxiety without side effects.[40] One experiment on dogs fed a diet fortified with caseinate hydrolysate showed significantly reduced signs of anxiety and plasma cortisol levels over 8 weeks.[41] A nutraceutical product primarily containing alpha-casozepine, has been shown to significantly reduce social anxiety in cats.[26] In another study, the same product was found to be equally as effective as selegiline and significantly improved emotional evaluation scores in dogs.[27]

In addition to the nutraceutical, there are 2 commercially available therapeutic diets containing alpha-casozepine. The first diet was fed to dogs before receiving nail trims and was found to reduce stranger-directed fear and aggression, nonsocial fear, and touch sensitivity during the procedure.[21] However, this study did not control for habituation, which may have accounted for some portion of the improved behavior. A feline formulation of the same diet was tested and found to decrease 2 indicators of anxiety in cats left alone in an unfamiliar room.[23] A more recently released diet containing alpha-casozepine has been shown to improve anxiety scores and help to reduce the signs associated with feline lower urinary tract disease.[20] It should be noted that these diets contain other functional ingredients, such as tryptophan, which may also contribute to their effectiveness.

Alpha-Lactalbumin

Similar to alpha-casozepine, alpha-lactalbumin is a bovine milk protein derivative. However, it is derived from the whey protein component of milk, not casein. Alpha-lactalbumin contains high concentrations of amino acids, including tryptophan.[42] It is believed that chronic anxiety depletes brain serotonin and its precursor, tryptophan, which can affect the ability to cope with further stressors[43] and performance on certain cognitive tasks.[44] The proposed rationale for the use of alpha-lactalbumin is that it replenishes stores of tryptophan and, therefore, will help to increase serotonin levels. This hypothesis was tested in human subjects by administering alpha-lactalbumin

Table 1
Functional ingredients found in specific behavioral nutraceuticals and therapeutic diets

Functional Ingredient	Nutraceutical	Therapeutic Diet
Alpha-casozepine	Zylkene (Vetoquinol, Fort Worth, TX)	Royal Canin Veterinary Diet Calm and Royal Canin Veterinary Diet Multifunction Urinary + Calm (Royal Canin USA, St. Charles, MO) Hill's Prescription Diet c/d Multicare Stress (Hill's Pet Nutrition, Topeka, KS)
Alpha-lactalbumin	Solliquin (Nutramax Laboratories, Lancaster, SC)	
Apoaequorin	Neutricks (Neutricks, Madison, WI)	
L-Theanine (Suntheanine)	Anxitane (Virbac Corporation, Fort Worth, TX) Composure and Composure PRO (VetriScience Laboratories, Williston, VT) Solliquin (Nutramax Laboratories)	
Magnolia officinalis and *Phellodendron amurense*	Solliquin (Nutramax Laboratories)	
Medium chain triglycerides		Purina Pro Plan Veterinary Diets NeuroCare and Purina Pro Plan Bright Mind (Nestle Purina Petcare Company, St. Louis, MO)
Omega 3 fatty acids		Hill's Prescription Diet b/d and Hill's Prescription Diet c/d Multicare Stress (Hill's Pet Nutrition, Topeka, KS) Purina Pro Plan Veterinary Diets NeuroCare (Nestle Purina Petcare Company)
S-Adenosylmethionine (SAMe)	Denosyl and Denamarin (Nutramax) Novifit (Virbac Corporation, Fort Worth, TX)	
Tryptophan	Composure PRO (VetriScience Laboratories, Williston, VT)	Hill's Prescription Diet c/d Multicare Stress (Hill's Pet Nutrition) Royal Canin Veterinary Diet Calm and Royal Canin Veterinary Diet Multifunction Urinary + Calm (Royal Canin USA)
Vitamin E, *Ginkgo biloba*, phosphatidylserine, resveratrol, and pyridoxine blend	Senilife (Ceva Animal Health, Lenexa, KS)	

Table 2
Common behavioral nutraceuticals, therapeutic diets, and associated product research (not including products for CDS)

Product Trade Name	Functional Ingredient(s)	Research Author(s)	Publication Type	Behavioral Condition	Target Species	Study Type	No. of Subjects	Parameters with Significant Positive Effects Attributable to Product
Anxitane	L-Theanine (Suntheanine)	Dramard et al,[9,10] 2007	Abstract[9] Proceedings[10]	Anxiety	Feline	Clinical trial, uncontrolled	33 test	Results reported with descriptive statistics only: 62% reduction in median global anxiety score (decreased anxiety) after 30 d[a]
		Berteselli & Michelazzi,[11,12] 2007	Abstract[11] Proceedings[12]	Noise and storm phobias	Canine	Clinical trial, controlled, did not specify if blinded or randomized	4 Tx + B-mod 3 B-mod only 4 nonphobic control	Decreased behavioral scores (decreased anxiety), hiding, and attention seeking in Tx + B-mod group after 60 d ($P<.05$)[b]
		Michelazzi et al,[13] 2010; Michelazzi et al,[14] 2015	Abstract[13] Journal[14]	Noise phobia	Canine	Clinical trial, placebo-controlled, randomized, did not specify if blinded	10 test 10 placebo	Decreased panting, yawning, drooling, drawing owner's attention, vocalizing, and compulsive behaviors compared with control ($P<.05$)[a]
		Araujo et al,[15] 2010	Journal	Fear of unfamiliar humans	Canine	Laboratory model, placebo-controlled, blinded, randomized	5 test 5 placebo	Longer time spent near human compared with control ($P = .0472$) Longer time interacting with human compared with control ($P = .0283$) Increased interaction frequency compared with control ($P = .0283$)
		Pike et al,[16] 2015	Journal	Storm sensitivity	Canine	Clinical trial, open label, uncontrolled	18 test	Decreased global anxiety score (decreased anxiety) ($P<.0001$) Decreased time to return to baseline normal behavior (faster recovery) ($P = .0063$)

(continued on next page)

Table 2
(continued)

Product Trade Name	Functional Ingredient(s)	Research Author(s)	Publication Type	Behavioral Condition	Target Species	Study Type	No. of Subjects	Parameters with Significant Positive Effects Attributable to Product
Composure	Thiamine C3 Colostrum-Calming complex L-Theanine (Suntheanine)	VetriScience Laboratories,[17] 2008	Unpublished	Various anxieties	Canine Feline	Clinical trial, case series, uncontrolled	10 cats 30 dogs	Results reported with descriptive statistics only: 79% effectiveness score in dogs, 73% effectiveness score in cats
	L-Theanine (Suntheanine)	VetriScience Laboratories,[18] 2016	Unpublished	Thunderstorm noise-induced anxiety	Canine	Laboratory model, controlled, blinded, did not specify if randomized	12 test 12 control	No statistical analysis reported: Less distance traveled (less anxiety) at 30 min and 4 h compared with control
Composure PRO	Thiamine L-Tryptophan C3 Colostrum-Calming Complex L-Theanine (Suntheanine)	No product research available						
Harmonease[c]	*Magnolia officinalis Phellodendron amurense*	DePorter et al,[19] 2012	Journal	Thunderstorm noise-induced anxiety	Canine	Laboratory model, placebo-controlled, crossover, blinded	20 dogs serving as their own control	Decreased inactivity duration (decreased anxiety) during thunderstorm noise phase in treatment group compared with baseline ($P<.03$) Increased distance traveled (reduced anxiety) in treatment group during thunderstorm noise phase compared with placebo ($P = .0565$)

Hill's Prescription Diet c/d Multicare Stress	Alpha-casozepine L-Tryptophan DHA EPA Antioxidants	Meyer & Becvarova,[20] 2016	Journal	FIC	Feline	Clinical trial, case series, uncontrolled	10 test	Improved QoL scores ($P>.05$) Improved emotional scores for contact with people and for other fears ($P<.05$) Improved FLUTD sign scores ($P<.05$) Improved overgrooming scores ($P<.05$)
Royal Canin Veterinary Diet Calm	Alpha-casozepine L-Tryptophan DHA EPA	Kato et al,[21] 2012	Journal	Anxiety-related behaviors	Canine	Clinical trial, controlled, crossover design, order not randomized	28 dogs serving as their own control	Improved scores for stranger-directed aggression ($P = .014$), stranger-directed fear ($P = .014$), nonsocial fear ($P = .031$), and touch sensitivity ($P<.001$) during nail trimming while receiving the test diet compared with control Poststressor UCCR increases from baseline were lower in dogs while receiving the test diet compared with placebo ($P = .04$)

(continued on next page)

Table 2
(continued)

Product Trade Name	Functional Ingredient(s)	Research Author(s)	Publication Type	Behavioral Condition	Target Species	Study Type	No. of Subjects	Parameters with Significant Positive Effects Attributable to Product
		Miyaji et al,[22] 2015	Journal	None	Feline	Clinical trial, controlled, randomized, blinded	10 test 11 control	Increased ratio of plasma tryptophan to LNAA from baseline after 8 wk compared with placebo (*P*<.05) Decreased urine cortisol concentration from baseline after 8 wk compared with placebo (*P*<.05)
		Landsberg et al,[23] 2017	Journal	Anxiety	Feline	Laboratory model, controlled, did not specify if blinded or randomized	12 test 12 control	Inactivity duration in an OFT did not significantly increase after 2 wk in test group (anxiety did not significantly worsen in unfamiliar location) (*P* = .07) compared with a significant increase in control group after 2 and 4 wk (*P*<.05) Increased inactivity frequency in an OFT (decreased anxiety in unfamiliar location) after 2 wk in test group (*P*<.05)
Solliquin	L-Theanine M officinalis P amurense Alpha-lactalbumin	DePorter et al,[24] 2016	Proceedings	Fear or anxiety	Canine Feline	Clinical trial, case series, open label, uncontrolled	15 dogs 1 cat	Results reported with descriptive statistics: 73.6% of subjects showed an effective response
		Landsberg et al,[25] 2017	Proceedings	Thunderstorm noise-induced anxiety	Canine	Laboratory model, placebo-controlled, randomized	14 test 14 placebo	Decreased distance traveled [reduced anxiety] in response to thunder from baseline to day 2 (*P* = .0284) Decreased inactivity frequency (reduced anxiety) from baseline to day 2 (*P* = .0435)

Zylkene	Alpha-casozepine	Beata et al,[26] 2007	Journal	Anxiety (social phobia)	Feline	Clinical trial, placebo-controlled, randomized, blinded	17 test 17 placebo	Increased scores (decreased anxiety) at day 56 for contact tolerance of familiar people ($P = .04$), contact tolerance of unfamiliar people ($P = .03$), and global emotional scores ($P = .003$)
		Beata et al,[27] 2007	Journal	Anxiety	Canine	Clinical trial, positive-controlled, randomized, blinded	19 test 19 selegiline control	Decreased EDED score from baseline (decreased anxiety) ($P>.0001$) Increased owner assessment score from baseline (decreased anxiety) ($P<.001$) No difference in treatment success (as equally effective as selegiline) based on EDED score ($P = .74$) and owner assessment ($P = .73$)

Abbreviations: B-mod, behavior modification; CDS, cognitive dysfunction syndrome; DHA, docosahexaenoic acid; EDED, emotional disorders evaluation in dogs; EPA, eicosapentaenoic acid; FIC, feline interstitial cystitis; FLUTD, feline lower urinary tract disease; LNAA, large neutral amino acids; OFT, open field test; QoL, quality of life; Tx, treatment; UCCR, urine cortisol creatinine ratio.

a *P* value was not reported in the published abstract but was given in the conference proceedings.
b *P* value was not reported in the conference proceedings but was given in the published abstract.
c Harmonease (Veterinary Products Laboratories, Phoenix, AZ) is no longer available.

Table 3
Common CDS nutraceuticals, therapeutic diets, and associated product research

Product Trade Name	Functional Ingredient(s)	Research Author(s)	Publication Type	Target Species	Design	No. of Subjects	Parameters with Significant Positive Effects Attributable to Product
Denamarin	SAMe Silybin	No product research related to behavioral use					
Denosyl	SAMe	No product research related to behavioral use					
Hill's Prescription Diet b/d	DHA EPA L-Carnitine Lipoic acid Vitamin C Vitamin E Carotenoids Flavonoids	Milgram et al,[28] 2002	Journal	Canine	Laboratory model, controlled, did not specify if blinded or randomized	12 aged test 11 aged control 9 young test 7 young control	Significant overall effect of diet on results of oddity discrimination learning tasks ($P = .0034$) Fewer errors (improved cognition) on 2 of 4 of the oddity discrimination learning tasks in aged dogs fed the test diet compared with aged controls ($P = .05$)
		Dodd et al,[29] 2002	Proceedings	Canine	Clinical trial, placebo-controlled, randomized, blinded	61 test 64 placebo	Increased interaction and activity after 60 d when compared with control ($P<.05$) Increased family recognition, animal recognition, and agility after 60 d when compared with control ($P<.05$)
		Milgram et al,[30] 2005	Journal	Canine	Laboratory model, placebo-controlled, did not specify if blinded or randomized	12 control diet + no enrichment 12 control diet + enrichment 12 test diet + no enrichment 12 test diet + enrichment	Improved performance (improved cognition) on black/white discrimination reversal learning task in dogs fed the test diet compared with control diet ($P<.05$)

Novifit	SAMe (NoviSAMe)	Reme et al,[31] 2008	Journal	Canine	Clinical trial, placebo-controlled, randomized, blinded	17 test 19 placebo	Greater improvement in activity scores at 4 wk (P<.003) and 8 wk (P<.03) compared with placebo Greater improvement in awareness scores at 4 wk (P<.05) and 8 wk (P<.01) compared with placebo
		Araujo et al,[32] 2012	Journal	Canine Feline	Laboratory model, placebo-controlled, randomized	7 test dogs 7 placebo dogs 8 test cats 8 placebo cats	Fewer errors (improved cognition) in treatment group compared with placebo in cats only (P = .015) Increased errors (decreased cognition) during reversal phase for control group compared with treatment in cats only (P = .003)
Neutricks	Apoaequorin	Milgram et al,[33] 2015	Journal	Canine	Study 1: Laboratory model, placebo-controlled, did not specify if blinded or randomized Study 2: Laboratory model, positive-controlled, did not specify if blinded or randomized	Study 1: (8) 2.5 mg dose (8) 5 mg dose 8 placebo Study 2: (8) 5-mg dose (8) 10-mg dose 8 selegiline	Study 1: Decreased number of errors (improved cognition) on discrimination task in 2.5-mg group compared with placebo (P = .04) Higher percent accuracy (improved cognition) on discrimination task in low-dose group compared with placebo (P = .03) Study 2: Increased performance accuracy (improved cognition) on attention task in 10 mg group compared with selegiline group when cognitive status and age were used as covariates (P<.01)

(continued on next page)

Table 3
(continued)

Product Trade Name	Functional Ingredient(s)	Research Author(s)	Publication Type	Target Species	Design	No. of Subjects	Parameters with Significant Positive Effects Attributable to Product
Purina Pro Plan Veterinary Diets NeuroCare	MCTs (6.5%), Arginine, DHA, EPA, Vitamins B_6 and B_9, Vitamin C, Vitamin E	Landsberg et al,[34] 2017	Proceedings	Canine	Clinical trial, placebo-controlled, randomized, did not specify if blinded	(29) 6.5% MCT (29) 9.0% MCT 29 placebo	Decreased scores (improved cognition) for disorientation, social interaction, sleep–wake cycle, house training, anxiety, and activity compared with baseline in dogs fed 6.5% MCT diet after 90 d ($P<.05$)
Purina Pro Plan Bright Mind	MCTs (5.5%), Arginine, DHA, EPA, Linoleic acid, Vitamins E and C, Pyridoxine	Pan et al,[35] 2010	Journal	Canine	Laboratory model, controlled, did not specify if blinded or randomized	12 test 12 control	Fewer errors (improved cognition) on landmark discrimination task compared with control ($P<.05$) Fewer errors (improved cognition) on reversal learning task compared with control ($P<.05$) Fewer errors (improved cognition) on complex landmark discrimination task compared with control ($P<.05$)
Senilife	Phosphatidylserine, Pyridoxine, Vitamin E, Ginkgo biloba extract, Resveratrol[a]	Osella et al,[36] 2007	Journal	Canine	Clinical trial, open-label, uncontrolled	8 test	Improved scores for disorientation, interaction, sleep–wake cycle, and activity from baseline to day 84 ($P<.001$)
		Araujo et al,[37] 2008	Journal	Canine	Laboratory model, placebo-controlled, cross-over design, randomized, blinded	9 dogs, serving as their own control	Improved DNMP test performance (improved short-term memory) from baseline ($P = .039$)

Abbreviations: CDS, cognitive dysfunction syndrome; DHA, docosahexaenoic acid; DNMP, delayed nonmatching to position; EPA, eicosapentaenoic acid; MCTs, medium chain triglycerides; SAMe, S-adenosylmethionine.

[a] When these studies were conducted, Senilife was formulated without resveratrol. The product composition has since been changed to include resveratrol.

to high-stress individuals and testing their performance on learning and memory.[45] The results showed that the subjects had a significant improvement in their cognitive tests after receiving the alpha-lactalbumin compared with their performance after a control diet.

Currently, there is only 1 veterinary behavioral nutraceutical containing alpha-lactalbumin. The product contains a key functional ingredient that is a proprietary whey protein concentrate rich in alpha-lactalbumin. In a case series report, pets given this nutraceutical showed a 74% effective response to treatment.[24] Additionally, a recent randomized, placebo-controlled study demonstrated decreased anxiety in dogs exposed to thunderstorm sounds after receiving the product for only 1 day.[25] As with other products, this nutraceutical contains multiple functional ingredients, and its effects cannot be attributed solely to alpha-lactalbumin.

Apoaequorin

Apoaequorin is a calcium-binding protein obtained from jellyfish. Intracellular calcium dysregulation associated with age is believed to contribute to the pathogenesis of Alzheimer's disease in humans.[46] It is proposed that apoaequorin acts as a calcium scavenger and reduces the effects of calcium dysregulation.[33] In vitro studies of apoaequorin have demonstrated the ability to reduce calcium-related neuronal cell death.[47] Clinically, apoaequorin was found to have direct beneficial cognitive effects in humans.[47] In aged beagle dogs, the apoaequorin was tested and shown to improve dogs' performance on learning and attention tasks more significantly than selegiline.[33]

L-Theanine

L-Theanine is an amino acid naturally found in tea plants that is thought to have several effects on the central nervous system. Theanine is suggested to increase GABA, serotonin, and dopamine levels in specific areas of the brain.[48,49] L-Theanine's structure is similar to that of glutamate, the major excitatory neurotransmitter, and will competitively bind to glutamate receptors, thereby blocking excitatory neurotransmission. This agent also serves a neuroprotective function by decreasing excessive glutamate, a known cause of neurotoxicity.[50] L-Theanine has been found to reduce physiologic and psychological stress responses in 1 study on humans, but it is unclear which neurotransmitter increase causes this effect.[51]

Most veterinary nutraceuticals containing L-theanine use a patented, purified form called Suntheanine (Taiyo International, Tokyo, Japan). Several studies have been performed on 1 particular veterinary nutraceutical product whose only functional ingredient is L-theanine. The most notable findings have been demonstrated in dogs, including a reduced fear of unfamiliar people,[15] reduced noise phobia,[11–14] and decreased storm-related anxiety.[16] One study on cats demonstrated a decrease in anxiety after 30 days of treatment.[9,10]

Magnolia officinalis and Phellodendron amurense

Extracts from the bark of *M officinalis* contain the active compounds honokiol and magnolol. These compounds have been demonstrated to bind $GABA_A$ receptors and enhance neurotransmission in vitro.[52] They have also been demonstrated to produce an anxiolytic effect in mice.[53] *P amurense* bark extracts contain the compound berberine that acts as a neuroprotective agent by blocking glutamate release.[54] Studies on combination products containing both *M officinalis* and *P amurense* have shown decreased salivary cortisol and improved mood scores in humans[55] and decreased thunderstorm noise-related anxiety in dogs.[19] The veterinary nutraceutical containing *M officinalis* and *P amurense* as the sole functional ingredients is no longer available. However, these ingredients are available in a newer combination product that also contains alpha-lactalbumin and L-theanine and has been shown to decrease anxiety.[24,25]

Medium Chain Triglycerides

The use of medium chain triglycerides (MCTs) is a relatively newer development in veterinary medicine and has been shown to be effective as an adjunctive treatment for canine idiopathic epilepsy and cognitive dysfunction syndrome.[34,35,56] In aging dogs, the brain's ability to metabolize glucose as an energy source decreases.[57] Diets with MCTs provide an alternative source of energy in the form of ketones.[35] In 1 study, aged beagles with decreased cognitive ability fed a diet containing 5.5% MCT for 8 months showed improved performance on cognitive tests.[35] A second diet with 6.5% MCT fed to privately owned dogs showed a significant improvement in clinical signs of cognitive dysfunction after 30 days.[34]

Melatonin

Melatonin is a hormone synthesized from serotonin in the pineal gland and secreted in maximal values during the night, consistent with the diurnal pattern of sleep–wake cycles. Melatonin is believed bind to $GABA_A$ receptors and may mimic the actions of benzodiazepines.[58] In dogs and cats, melatonin is purported to be of use for the treatment of sleep–wake cycle disturbances, anxiety, and fear,[7] but scientific evidence is lacking. There is 1 published case report that describes rapid improvement in a dog with noise and thunderstorm phobias when treated with a combination of amitriptyline, melatonin, and behavioral modification.[59]

Omega-3 Fatty Acids

Omega-3 fatty acids (also written as n-3 fatty acids) are long-chain polyunsaturated fatty acids considered to be essential to the diets of mammals. Dietary sources of the omega-3 fatty acids docosahexaenoic acid (DHA) and eicosapentaenoic acid (EPA) mainly originate from fish oils.[60] DHA has been shown to play a vital role in the development of neural and retinal tissue of puppies[61] as well as cognitive learning, memory,[8] and trainability.[62] These studies suggest the importance of feeding diets fortified with DHA to dams during gestation and lactation and to puppies after weaning. EPA's value has been better demonstrated as an antiinflammatory agent.[63] In aged dogs, a diet containing DHA and EPA was shown to reduce signs of age-associated cognitive decline and improve learning.[28–30] However, these diets were also rich in antioxidants and mitochondrial cofactors and contained relatively low amounts of DHA and EPA.[64] This factor suggests that the findings may be more attributable to the antioxidants and mitochondrial cofactors. One study found that aggressive German shepherd dogs had lower plasma DHA and a higher omega-6 to omega-3 ratio compared with nonaggressive controls.[65] However, this study did not control for diet composition among subjects. Regardless, the results show only correlation and not causation. No studies demonstrate the effects of fatty acid supplementation on aggressive dogs or cats.

S-Adenosylmethionine

S-Adenosylmethionine (SAMe) exists in all living cells. It plays a critical role in cellular metabolism and contributes to maintaining cell membranes, the synthesis and inactivation of neurotransmitters (including norepinephrine, dopamine, and serotonin), and the synthesis of glutathione (an important cellular antioxidant).[66] Reduced levels of SAMe have been found in the brains of human patients with Alzheimer's disease.[67]

Although this finding has not been evaluated in canines, there are multiple other parallels in brain pathology between Alzheimer's disease and canine cognitive dysfunction, such as the accumulation of beta-amyloid plaques.[68] In a laboratory study, dogs and cats with cognitive dysfunction syndrome given SAMe showed improved cognitive abilities.[32] One clinical study reported senior dogs treated with SAMe showed improvements in activity and awareness, which are commonly affected by cognitive dysfunction.[31]

Tryptophan

Tryptophan is another dietary amino acid used in the management of behavioral conditions. It is converted to 5-hydroxytryptophan, which is the rate-limiting step in the production of serotonin. The availability of tryptophan largely depends on diet. Not only is the amount of tryptophan important, the ratio of tryptophan to other large neutral amino acids (LNAAs) is also significant.[69] Dietary protein contains larger proportions of LNAAs compared with tryptophan. These LNAAs compete with tryptophan for access to the carrier protein that transports them across the blood–brain barrier, where serotonin is made.[70] High protein meals are likely to decrease the availability of tryptophan to the brain due to the increased ratio of LNAAs.[71] This may explain why 1 study found that dogs fed a high protein diet had higher scores for owner-directed aggression (previously referred to as "dominance aggression") than other test groups.[72] The same study also reported that territorial behavior scores were lower when fed a diet with low protein and tryptophan supplementation. Research has been conducted on plasma tryptophan and LNAA levels. One study found decreased plasma tryptophan and increased tryptophan metabolites in fearful dogs, suggesting a correlation between tryptophan metabolism and fear.[73] In another study, tryptophan supplementation in mildly anxious dogs increased plasma tryptophan and tryptophan to LNAA ratios, but did not cause any significant changes in behavior.[74] In clinical research, 2 studies were able to demonstrate a reduction of stress-related behaviors attributable to tryptophan supplementation in cats and working dogs.[75,76] There is no veterinary behavioral nutraceutical that contains tryptophan alone. However, some nutraceuticals and therapeutic diets contain tryptophan in additional to other functional ingredients.

Other Functional Ingredients

Antioxidants
Several antioxidants, such as alpha-tocopherol (vitamin E), ascorbic acid (vitamin C), carotenoids (including beta-carotene), flavonoids, long chain polyunsaturated fatty acids, *Ginkgo biloba*, and resveratrol are used in some of the veterinary behavior nutraceuticals or therapeutic diets. These substances combat the effects of oxidative stress, which cause some of the neurodegenerative changes seen in cognitive dysfunction.[37]

Phosphatidylserine
Phosphatidylserine is a phospholipid associated with proteins that regulate neural membrane fluidity.[77]

Pyridoxine (vitamin B_6)
Pyridoxine is a vital cofactor in the synthesis of neurotransmitters, including serotonin.[77]

Mitochondrial cofactors
Both alpha-lipoic acid and L-carnitine are used in mitochondrial functions. Alpha-lipoic acid contributes to the mitochondrial processes that recycle antioxidants and increase

glutathione. Chronic oxidative damage can reduce the metabolic capacity of mitochondria. Supplementation of these cofactor increases their concentration and can restore mitochondrial efficiency.[78]

Trace minerals

Trace minerals such as selenium, zinc, copper, and manganese can act as free radical scavengers or help to recycle antioxidants.[78]

CLINICAL APPLICATION
When to Use Nutraceuticals or Therapeutic Diets

Once a veterinarian has reviewed a nutraceutical or therapeutic diet and its associated literature, they will then need to decide when the use of that product is appropriate. As always, a thorough physical examination and screening laboratory work should be performed to rule out any medical conditions contributing to a behavioral diagnosis. After a diagnostic work-up, an accurate behavioral diagnosis is needed. Also crucial in the treatment plan of any behavioral condition is the inclusion of behavior modification and environmental management. Nutraceuticals and therapeutic diets (or medication for that matter) should not be the only recommendations given to clients. Nutraceuticals and therapeutic diets are certainly suitable for the treatment of mild behavioral conditions, especially for early intervention to prevent the condition from worsening.[77] But for more advanced cases, a psychopharmacologic agent may be the more appropriate choice. Some nutraceuticals or therapeutic diets can be used as adjunctive treatments to medications. However, attention to the functional ingredient's mode of action and any risk for interaction with a pharmacologic agent should be investigated before combining treatments. This point is especially important when prescribing serotonergic medications together with functional ingredients that also increase serotonin. It may be the safest practice to avoid these combinations altogether, particularly for prescribers who are inexperienced with behavior-modifying agents. Clients should always be advised to monitor their pets for adverse reactions when prescribing nutraceuticals, therapeutic diets, and when using combination therapies.

Patient and Client Needs

There may be times when the use of a nutraceutical or therapeutic diet will have its advantages over medications. These modes of treatment can come in more palatable forms than some medications. Certain drug options can be bitter in taste, which can make medicating the pet difficult for owners. Pets who are not treat motivated may be more likely to eat a therapeutic diet than take a nutraceutical in chewable tablet form or a pill wrapped in human food. An important component in the treatment of any behavioral condition is to decrease the patient's overall anxiety and avoid any confrontational interactions with the pet. If pilling a pet will cause unnecessary stress or damage to the human–animal bond, then choosing an alternative treatment may be the best option. (There are also methods for using positive reinforcement to train a pet to take medications, but that goes beyond the scope of this article.) Struggling with the pet to medicate it not only decreases the quality of life for both the patient and owner, but also reduces the chance of compliance with your treatment plan and likelihood of success.

Another obstacle to treatment can be the stigma people often associate with mental illness. In human medicine, it is not uncommon for people to have a negative opinion of psychotropic medication.[79] This belief can be projected onto pets and affect what treatments clients are willing to pursue. Despite appropriate education from the veterinarian, clients may still be reluctant to start their pet on behavioral medications. In these cases, the use of a "natural" nutraceutical or therapeutic diet may be perfectly acceptable to the client. There are other times when clients may simply not be ready to accept the idea that their pet needs medication to treat their behavioral condition. A nutraceutical or therapeutic diet may serve as a compromise when discussing the treatment plan with the client. If the pet's behavior has not improved after 1 to 2 months of treatment, then you may be able to revisit the discussion of using a medication. For these cases, the nutraceutical or therapeutic diet may serve as a sort of "gateway drug" before the client will accept the idea of implementing a psychopharmacologic agent for their pet.

Unfortunately, financial constraints may play a role in deciding a treatment option. Many nutraceuticals and therapeutic diets can be understandably costly, especially for large breed dogs. Caution should be exercised to ensure a client will not seek out less expensive, over-the-counter, human versions of nutraceuticals because these products may be lesser in quality, contain unsafe dosages of ingredients, or contain potentially harmful ingredients (eg, xylitol). If a client is unable or unwilling to pay for a higher priced treatment, it may be more feasible to prescribe an extralabel medication (if medically appropriate) that is available in generic form at a more manageable cost.

It is important for veterinarians to discuss therapeutic options with clients before prescribing treatment. This step will help to determine the option with which clients are most likely to comply. After initiating a treatment plan, follow-up with the client is vital. Close monitoring is necessary to gauge response to treatment and determine whether adjustments need to be made.

REFERENCES

1. Boothe DM. Nutraceuticals: must or myth? In: CVC San Diego Proceedings. 2010. Available at: http://veterinarycalendar.dvm360.com/nutraceuticals-myth-or-must-proceedings. Accessed October 14, 2017.

2. Title 21 United States Code Section 321. 2017. Available at: http://uscode.house.gov/view.xhtml?req=granuleid:USC-prelim-title21-section321&num=0&edition=prelim. Accessed October 14, 2017.

3. Dzanis DA. Nutraceutical and dietary supplements. In: Fascetti AJ, Delaney SJ, editors. Applied veterinary clinical nutrition. 1st edition. Ames (IA): John Wiley & Sons, Inc; 2012. p. 57–67.

4. Boothe DM. Nutraceuticals in veterinary medicine, part 1: definitions and regulations. Compend Contin Educ Vet 1997;19:1248–55.

5. University of Oxford. Oxford Centre for evidence-based medicine – Levels of evidence (March 2009). 2009. Available at: http://www.cebm.net/oxford-centre-evidence-based-medicine-levels-evidence-march-2009/. Accessed October 14, 2017.

6. Keene BW. Editorial: towards evidence-based veterinary medicine. J Vet Intern Med 2000;14:118–9.

7. Landsberg G, Hunthausen W, Ackerman L. Complimentary and alternative therapy for behavior problems. In: Behavior problems of the dog and cat. 3rd edition. Philadelphia: Saunders Elsevier; 2013. p. 139–49.

8. Zicker SC, Jewell DE, Yamka RM, et al. Evaluation of cognitive learning, memory, psychomotor, immunologic, and retinal functions in healthy puppies fed foods fortified with docosahexaenoic acid-rich fish oil from 8 to 52 weeks of age. J Am Vet Med Assoc 2012;241:583–94.

9. Dramard V, Kern L, Hofmans J, et al. Clinical efficacy of l-theanine tablets to reduce anxiety-related emotional disorders in cats: a pilot open-label clinical trial [abstract]. J Vet Behav 2007;2:85–6.

10. Dramard V, Kern L, Hofmans J, et al. Clinical efficacy of l-theanine tablets to reduce anxiety-related emotional disorders in cats: a pilot open-label clinical trial. In: Proceedings of the 6th International Veterinary Behavior Conference. Riccione (Italy), June 17–20, 2007.

11. Berteselli GV, Michelazzi M. Use of l-theanine tablets (Anxitane) and behaviour modification for treatment of phobias in dogs: a preliminary study [abstract]. J Vet Behav 2007;2:101.

12. Berteselli GV, Michelazzi M. Use of l-theanine tablets and behavior modification for treatment of phobias in dogs: a preliminary study. In: Proceedings of the 6th International Veterinary Behavior Conference. Riccione (Italy), June 17–20, 2007.

13. Michelazzi M, Berteselli G, Minero M, et al. Effectiveness of l-theanine and behavioral therapy in the treatment of noise phobias in dogs [abstract]. J Vet Behav 2010;5:34–5.

14. Michelazzi M, Berteselli GV, Talamonti Z, et al. Efficacy of l-theanine in the treatment of noise phobias in dogs: preliminary results. Veterinaria 2015;29:53–9.

15. Araujo JA, de Rivera C, Ethier JL, et al. Anxitane tablets reduce fear of human beings in a laboratory model of anxiety-related behavior. J Vet Behav 2010;5:268–75.

16. Pike AL, Horwitz DF, Lobprise H. An open-label prospective study of the use of l-theanine (Anxitane) in storm-sensitive client-owned dogs. J Vet Behav 2015;10:324–31.

17. Vetriscience Laboratories. Field trial of Composure products. Available at: http://resources.vet-advantage.com/media/attachments/2015/02/03/VSD53_Compos_Clinical.pdf. Accessed October 14, 2017.

18. Vetriscience Laboratories. Assessment of anxiolytic properties of a novel compound in beagle dogs with a noise-induced model of fear and anxiety. Available at: http://vetriproline.com/composure-pro/. Accessed October 14, 2017.

19. DePorter TL, Landsberg GM, Araujo JL, et al. Harmonease reduces noise-induced fear and anxiety in a laboratory canine model of thunderstorm simulation: a blinded and placebo-controlled study. J Vet Behav 2012;7:225–32.

20. Meyer HP, Becvarova I. Effects of a urinary food supplemented with milk protein hydrolysate and l-tryptophan on feline idiopathic cystitis – results of a case series in 10 cats. Int J Appl Res Vet Med 2016;14:59–65.

21. Kato M, Miyaji K, Ohtani N, et al. Effects of prescription diet on dealing with stressful situations and performance of anxiety-related behaviors in privately owned anxious dogs. J Vet Behav 2012;7:21–6.

22. Miyaji K, Kato M, Ohtani N, et al. Experimental verification of the effects on normal domestic cats by feeding prescription diet for decreasing stress. J Appl Anim Welf Sci 2015;18:355–62.

23. Landsberg G, Milgram B, Mougeot I, et al. Therapeutic effects of an alpha-casozepine and L-tryptophan supplemented diet on fear and anxiety in the cat. J Feline Med Surg 2017;19:594–602.

24. DePorter TL, Bledsoe DL, Conley JR, et al. Case report series of clinical effectiveness and safety of Solliquin for behavioral support in dogs and cats. In: Veterinary Behavior Symposium Proceedings. San Antonio (TX), August 5, 2016. p. 27–8.

25. Landsberg G, Huggins S, Fish J, et al. The effects of a nutritional supplement (Solliquin) in reducing fear and anxiety in a laboratory model of thunder induced fear and anxiety. In: Veterinary Behavior Symposium Proceedings. Indianapolis (IN), July 20, 2017. p. 24–6.

26. Beata C, Beaumont-Graff E, Coll C, et al. Effect of alpha-casozepine (Zylkene) on anxiety in cats. J Vet Behav 2007;2:40–6.

27. Beata C, Beaumont-Graff E, Diaz C, et al. Effect of alpha-casozepine (Zylkene) versus selegiline hydrochloride (Selgian, Anipryl) on anxiety disorders in dogs. J Vet Behav 2007;2:175–83.

28. Milgram NW, Zicker SC, Head E, et al. Dietary enrichment counteracts age-associated cognitive dysfunction in canines. Neurobiol Aging 2002;23: 737–45.

29. Dodd CE, Zicker SC, Lowry SR, et al. Effects of an investigational food on age-related behavioral changes in dogs. In: Proceedings of the Symposium on Brain Aging and Related Behavioral Changes in Dogs. Orlando (FL), January 11, 2002.

30. Milgram NW, Head E, Zicker SC, et al. Learning ability in aged Beagle dogs is preserved by behavioral enrichment and dietary fortification: a two-year longitudinal study. Neurobiol Aging 2005;26:77–90.

31. Reme CA, Dramard V, Kern L, et al. Effect of S-adenosylmethionine tablets on the reduction of age-related mental decline in dogs: a double-blinded, placebo-controlled trial. Vet Ther 2008;9:69–82.

32. Araujo JA, Faubert ML, Brooks ML, et al. Novifit (SAMe) tablets improve executive function in aged dogs and cats: implications for treatment of cognitive dysfunction syndrome. Int J Appl Res Vet Med 2012;10:90–8.

33. Milgram NW, Landsberg G, Merrick D, et al. A novel mechanism for cognitive enhancement in aged dogs with the use of a calcium-buffering protein. J Vet Behav 2015;10:217–22.

34. Landsberg G, Pan Y, Mouget I, et al. Efficacy of a therapeutic diet on dogs with cognitive dysfunction syndrome. In: Veterinary Behavior Symposium Proceedings. Indianapolis (IN), July 20, 2017. p. 16.

35. Pan Y, Larson B, Araujo JA, et al. Dietary supplementation with medium-chain TAG has long-lasting cognition-enhancing effects in aged dogs. Br J Nutr 2010;103:1746–54.

36. Osella MC, Re G, Odore R, et al. Canine cognitive dysfunction syndrome: prevalence, clinical signs and treatment with a neuroprotective nutraceutical. Appl Anim Behav Sci 2007;105:297–310.

37. Araujo JA, Landsberg GM, Milgram NW, et al. Improvement of short-term memory performance in aged beagles by a nutraceutical supplement containing phosphatidylserine. Ginkgo biloba, vitamin E, and pyridoxine. Can Vet J 2008;49: 379–85.

38. Lecouvey M, Frochot C, Miclo L, et al. Two-dimensional 1H-NMR and CD structural analysis in a micellar medium of a bovine αs1-casein fragment having benzodiazepine-like properties. Eur J Biochem 1997;248:872–8.

39. Messaoudi M, Lalonde R, Schroeder H, et al. Anxiolytic-like effects and safety profile of a tryptic hydrolysate from bovine alpha s1-casein in rats. Fundam Clin Pharmacol 2009;23:323–30.

40. Violle N, Messaoudi M, Lefranc-Millot C, et al. Ethological comparison of the effects of a bovine alpha s1-casein tryptic hydrolysate and diazepam on the behavior of rats in two models an anxiety. Pharmacol Biochem Behav 2006;84: 517–23.

41. Palestrini C, Minero M, Cannas S, et al. Efficacy of a diet containing caseinate hydrolysate on sings of stress in dogs. J Vet Behav 2010;5:309–17.

42. Yalcin AS. Emerging therapeutic potential of whey proteins and peptides. Curr Pharm Des 2006;12:1637–43.

43. Adell A, Garcia-Marquez C, Armario A, et al. Chronic stress increases serotonin and noradrenaline in rat brain and sensitizes their responses to a further acute stress. J Neurochem 1998;50:1678–81.

44. Brand N, Jolles J. Information processing in depression and anxiety. Psychol Med 1987;17:145–53.

45. Markus CR, Olivier B, de Haan EH. Whey protein rich in alpha-lactalbumin increases the ratio of plasma tryptophan to the sum of the other large neutral amino acids and improves cognitive performance in stress-vulnerable subjects. Am J Clin Nutr 2002;75:1051–6.

46. Supnet C, Bezprozvanny I. The dysregulation of intracellular calcium in Alzheimer disease. Cell Calcium 2010;47:183–9.

47. Underwood M, Sivesind P, Gabourie T, et al. Effect of apoaequorin on cognitive function [abstract]. Alzheimers Dement 2011;7(suppl):e65.

48. Kimura R, Murata T. Influence of alkylamides of glutamic acid and related compounds on the central nervous system. I. Central depressant effect of theanine. Chem Pharm Bull 1971;19:1257–61.

49. Yokogoshi H, Kobayashi M, Mochizuki M, et al. Effect of theanine, r-glutamylethylamide, on brain monoamines and striatal dopamine release in conscious rats. Neurochem Res 1998;23:667–73.

50. Kakuda T, Nozawa A, Sugimoto A, et al. Inhibition by theanine of binding of [3H] AMPA,[3H] kainate, and [3H] MDL 105,519 to glutamate receptors. Biosci Biotechnol Biochem 2002;66:2683–6.

51. Kimura K, Ozeki M, Juneja LR, et al. L-Theanine reduces psychological and physiological stress responses. Biol Psychol 2007;74:39–45.

52. Alexeev M, Grosenbaugh DK, Mott DD, et al. The natural products magnolol and honokiol are positive allosteric modulators of both synaptic and extra-synaptic $GABA_A$ receptors. Neuropharmacology 2012;62:2507–14.

53. Maruyama Y, Kuribara H, Morita M, et al. Identification of magnolol and honokiol as anxiolytic agents in extracts of Saiboku-to, an oriental herbal medicine. J Nat Prod 1998;61:135–8.

54. Lin TY, Lin YW, Lu CW, et al. Berberine inhibits the release of glutamate in nerve terminals from rat cerebral cortex. PLoS One 2013;8:e67215.

55. Talbott SM, Talbott JA, Pugh M. Effect of *Magnolia officinalis* and *Phellodendron amurense* (Relora) on cortisol and psychological mood state in moderately stressed subjects. J Int Soc Sports Nutr 2013;10:37.

56. Law TH, Davies ES, Pan Y, et al. A randomised trial of a medium-chain TAG diet as treatment for dogs with idiopathic epilepsy. Br J Nutr 2015;114:1438–47.

57. London ED, Ohata M, Takei H, et al. Regional cerebral metabolic rate for glucose in beagle dogs of different ages. Neurobiol Aging 1983;4:121–6.

58. Golombek DA, Pevet P, Cardinali DP. Melatonin effect on behavior: possible mediation by the central GABAergic system. Neurosci Biobehav Rev 1996;20:406–12.

59. Aronson L. Animal behavior case of the month. J Am Vet Med Assoc 1999;215:22–4.

60. Lenox CE. An overview of fatty acids in companion animal medicine. J Am Vet Med Assoc 2015;246:1198–202.

61. Heinemann KM, Waldron MK, Bigley KE, et al. Long-chain (n-3) polyunsaturated fatty acids are more efficient than alpha-linolenic acid in improving electroretinogram responses of puppies exposed during gestation, lactation and weaning. J Nutr 2005;135:1960–6.

62. Kelley R, Lepine A, Morgan D. Improving puppy trainability through nutrition. In: Proceedings of the Societa Culturale Italiana Veterinari per Animali da Compagnia 56th International Congress. 2007. Available at: http://www.ivis.org/proceedings/scivac/2005/Morgan1_en.pdf?LA=1. Accessed October 14, 2017.
63. Logas D, Kunkle GA. Double-blinded crossover study with marine oil supplementation containing high dose eicosapentaenoic acid for the treatment of canine pruritic skin disease. Vet Dermatol 1994;5:99–104.
64. Bauer JE. The essential nature of dietary omega-3 fatty acids in dogs. J Am Vet Med Assoc 2016;249:1267–71.
65. Re S, Zanoletti M, Emanuele E. Aggressive dogs are characterized by low omega-3 polyunsaturated fatty acid status. Vet Res Commun 2008;32:225–30.
66. Bottiglieri T. S-adenosyl-L-methionine (SAMe): from the bench to the bedside – molecular basis of a pleiotrophic molecule. Am J Clin Nutr 2002;76(suppl):1151S–7S.
67. Morrison LD, Smith DD, Kish SJ. Brain S-adenosylmethionine levels are severely decreased in Alzheimer's disease. J Neurochem 1996;67:1328–31.
68. Cummings BJ, Su JH, Cottman CW, et al. Beta-amyloid accumulation in aged canine brain: a model of early plaque formation in Alzheimer's disease. Neurobiol Aging 1993;14:547–60.
69. Bosch G, Beerda B, Hendriks WH, et al. Impact of nutrition on canine behaviour: current status and possible mechanisms. Nutr Res Rev 2007;20:180–94.
70. Fernstrom JD, Wurtman RJ. Brain serotonin content: physiological regulation by plasma neutral amino acids. Science 1972;178:149–52.
71. Leathwood PD. Tryptophan availability and serotonin synthesis. Proc Nutr Soc 1987;46:143–56.
72. DeNapoli JS, Dodman NH, Shuster L, et al. Effect of dietary protein content and tryptophan supplementation on dominance aggression, territorial aggression, and hyperactivity in dogs. J Am Vet Med Assoc 2000;217:504–8.
73. Puurunen J, Tiira K, Lehtonen M, et al. Non-targeted metabolite profiling reveals changes in oxidative stress, tryptophan and lipid metabolisms in fearful dogs. Behav Brain Funct 2016;12:7.
74. Bosch G, Beerda B, Beynen AC, et al. Dietary tryptophan supplementation in privately owned mildly anxious dogs. Appl Anim Behav Sci 2009;121:197–205.
75. Pereira GG, Fragoso S, Pires E. Effect of dietary intake of L-tryptophan supplementation on multi-housed cats presenting stress related behaviours. In: Proceedings of the 53rd BSAVA Congress. Birmingham (UK), April 8–11, 2010.
76. Pereira GG, Fragoso S, Pires E. Effect of dietary intake of L-tryptophan supplementation on working dogs demonstrating stress related behaviours. In: Proceedings of the 53rd BSAVA Congress. Birmingham (UK), April 8–11, 2010.
77. Overall KL. Pharmacological approaches to changing behavior and neurochemistry: roles for diet, supplements, nutraceuticals, and medication. In: Manual of clinical behavioral medicine for dogs and cats. St Louis (MO): Elsevier Mosby; 2013. p. 458–512.
78. Zicker SC, Overall KL. Possible implications of oxidative stress in clinical veterinary behavioral medicine. Proceedings from the scientific symposium of the American Veterinary Society of Animal Behavior. Nashville (TN), July 12, 2002.
79. Jorm AF. Mental health literacy: public knowledge and beliefs about mental disorders. Br J Psychiatry 2000;177:396–401.

Printed and bound by CPI Group (UK) Ltd, Croydon, CR0 4YY

03/10/2024

01040393-0014